Advances in Burn Injuries - Physiology, Treatment, and Recovery

Edited by Selda Pelin Kartal

Published in London, United Kingdom

Advances in Burn Injuries - Physiology, Treatment, and Recovery
http://dx.doi.org/10.5772/intechopen.1012131
Edited by Selda Pelin Kartal

Contributors
Alhan Fernando, Andrew C. Bright, Ayşe Büşra Pekal, Chandler Hinson, Chow A. M. Roberta, Desmond Khor, Diroji Antony, Emily Vanderpool, Kevin Slaughter, Kimberly A. Donnellan, Kubilay Gürünlüoğlu, Maysa Shemmiyeva, Mehmet Demircan, Necmettin Akpinar, Nooshafarin Kazemikhoo, Ovunc Akdemir, Ozan Barıs Namdaroglu, Selda Pelin Kartal, Selen Ozturk, Shingo E. Yasuhara, Takahiko Tamura, Tunahan İnan, Tuğrul Çiçek, Yücel Pekal, Zerong You

First published in London, United Kingdom, 2026 by IntechOpen
IntechOpen is the global imprint of INTECHOPEN LIMITED, registered in England and Wales, registration number: 11086078, 167-169 Great Portland Street, London, W1W 5PF, United Kingdom

For EU product safety concerns: IN TECH d.o.o., Prolaz Marije Krucifikse Kozulić 3, 51000 Rijeka, Croatia, info@intechopen.com or visit our website at intechopen.com.

British Library Cataloguing-in-Publication Data
A catalogue record for this book is available from the British Library

Advances in Burn Injuries - Physiology, Treatment, and Recovery
Edited by Selda Pelin Kartal
p. cm.
Print ISBN 978-1-80631-772-1
Online ISBN 978-1-80631-771-4
eBook (PDF) ISBN 978-1-80631-773-8

Meet the editor

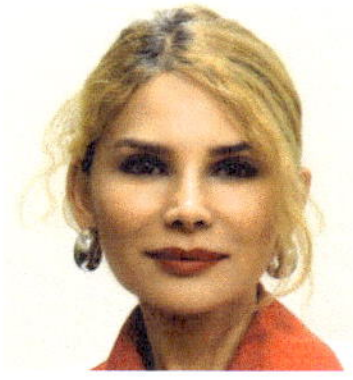

Selda Pelin Kartal graduated from Hacettepe University School of Medicine. She is currently a Professor and Head of the Department of Dermatology at the University of Health Sciences, Ministry of Health, Etlik City Hospital, Ankara, Turkey. She has co-authored over 200 published articles and supervised several master's and postdoctoral students. Her actual interests are acne, psoriasis, urticaria, autoimmune bullous diseases, Behçet's disease, and cosmetic dermatology.

Contents

Preface

Burn injuries remain one of the most challenging forms of trauma. Despite significant advances in prevention, critical care, surgical techniques, wound management, and rehabilitation, burn injuries continue to be associated with substantial morbidity, long-term disability, and profound psychosocial and economic consequences. Effective burn care requires a multidisciplinary approach that integrates fundamental biological knowledge with evidence-based clinical management and emerging therapeutic innovations.

This edited volume has been developed to provide readers with a comprehensive and contemporary perspective on burn injury. The volume opens with "Pathophysiology of Burn Damage", which provides an overview of the biological and physiological processes initiated by burn injury. This is followed by "Pathophysiology-Driven Treatment Strategies in Burn Injury", highlighting how an improved understanding of burn biology can guide therapeutic decision-making.

The section addressing systemic responses and consequences of burn injury includes "Nutrition in Burn Patients", which discusses the critical role of nutritional support in recovery and rehabilitation. The chapter entitled "Autophagy/Mitophagy Dysregulation and Neuroimmune Crosstalk in Burn-Induced Skeletal Muscle Dysfunction: Mechanistic Insights and Therapeutic Prospects" explores molecular mechanisms underlying burn-induced muscle dysfunction and their potential therapeutic implications.

Special clinical considerations are presented in "Burn Management in Children and Newborns", which examines the treatment of pediatric burn patients, and "Electrical Burn", which addresses the distinctive mechanisms, clinical manifestations, and management principles associated with electrical injuries.

Advances in wound care and regenerative therapies are discussed in "Wound Healing with Modern Burn Dressing with a Focus on Synthetic Polylactic Acid Membrane as the Best Example", which reviews modern dressing technologies and their role in tissue repair. This is followed by "Using Photobiomodulation in Treating Burn Ulcers", which examines the emerging role of light-based therapies in enhancing wound healing and regeneration.

The volume concludes with two chapters dedicated to long-term outcomes and sequelae of burn injury. "Comprehensive Approaches to Burn Scar Management" reviews current strategies for preventing and treating burn scars, whereas "Cutaneous Sequelae After Burn Injury: Pruritus, Dyspigmentation and Malignancy—Mechanisms and Management" addresses important dermatological complications that may arise during long-term follow-up.

We hope that this volume will serve as a valuable resource for clinicians, surgeons, researchers, trainees, and allied healthcare professionals involved in the care of burn patients. By bringing together current knowledge spanning basic mechanisms, clinical management, regenerative therapies, and long-term outcomes, this book aims to advance burn care and improve patient outcomes.

I'm grateful to all the contributors and leading experts for submitting their wonderful work, which provides an in-depth view of all aspects of the content, backed by the most current literature in the field. I offer special thanks to Publishing Process Mirna Papuga for bringing the book to its present form, and to my son Demir Durmazlar and Ares for their understanding of missed family time.

Prof. Dr. Selda Pelin Kartal
University of Health Science,
Department of Dermatology and Venereology,
Ministry of Health Etlik City Hospital,
Ankara, Turkey

Section 1

Basic Mechanisms of Burn Injury

Chapter 1

Pathophysiology of Burn Damage

Alhan Fernando

Abstract

Burn injury is a time-dependent disease process in which local tissue destruction and loss of barrier function rapidly trigger systemic derangements that shape clinical outcomes. The magnitude of injury is determined by the agent, temperature, and duration of exposure and is further modified by burn size and depth, inhalation injury, associated trauma, comorbidities, and delays to definitive care. At the wound level, thermal injury produces a heterogeneous pattern of damage classically described as concentric zones of coagulation, stasis, and hyperemia. This zonal organization is clinically important because the ischemic zone of stasis remains vulnerable to early progression, and cellular responses evolve over hours to days through overlapping pathways that include oxidative stress, autophagy, and apoptosis. Simultaneously, microvascular dysfunction and extracellular matrix disruption increase capillary permeability and impair interstitial restraint, promoting rapid fluid extravasation and progressive edema that compromises perfusion and contributes to burn shock physiology. Beyond the wound, severe burns induce a biphasic metabolic response, transitioning from an early hypometabolic period to a prolonged hypermetabolic state driven by sustained neuroendocrine activation and inflammatory signaling. In parallel, innate immune activation through danger and pathogen sensing amplifies cytokine networks and contributes to immune imbalance, predisposing to infection, sepsis, and multiple organ dysfunction. This chapter integrates these mechanisms to provide a coherent framework linking early local events to systemic failure, highlighting key biologic pathways that influence resuscitation, wound progression, and organ outcomes after severe burn trauma.

Keywords: burn, pathophysiology, hypermetabolism, damage-associated molecular patterns, necrosis

1. Introduction

Burn injury is not merely a localized cutaneous insult; it is a time-dependent, multi-scale disease process that begins at the moment of energy transfer and can evolve into a sustained systemic syndrome. For clinicians in plastic and reconstructive surgery, this dual nature is central: The same injury that destroys the skin's barrier and soft-tissue architecture also initiates microvascular failure, immune dysregulation, and profound metabolic stress that directly influence wound progression, timing of excision and grafting, susceptibility to infection, and ultimately the quality of long-term reconstruction. Understanding burn pathophysiology, therefore, provides the clinical "bridge" between early resuscitation and definitive coverage and between acute survival and functional, aesthetic recovery.

At the wound level, the Jackson model describes three concentric zones: coagulation (irreversible necrosis), stasis (hypoperfused but potentially salvageable tissue vulnerable to "burn wound conversion"), and hyperemia (reactive vasodilation with expected recovery). Early after major burns, microvascular permeability increases, producing capillary leak and edema that impair perfusion and oxygen delivery and contribute to burn shock physiology. In parallel, severe burns trigger a sustained hypermetabolic flow state driven by neuroendocrine stress and inflammatory mediators, causing insulin resistance, muscle wasting, and organ strain – effects that can persist long after the acute phase. Finally, tissue injury releases damage-associated molecular patterns (DAMPs) (and, when infection occurs, pathogen-associated molecular patterns [PAMPs]) that activate innate immune pathways (e.g., Toll-like receptors [TLR] signaling), shaping both systemic inflammation and later immune dysfunction that predispose to sepsis and multiple organ dysfunction syndromes (MODS) [1].

This chapter synthesizes these core mechanisms – zonal wound biology, microvascular failure, hypermetabolism, and innate immune activation – and links them to organ dysfunction and reconstructive outcomes, providing a practical pathophysiologic framework.

2. Mechanism of immediate tissue damage

Burn injuries produce structural and functional alterations across the different layers of the skin, as well as in the underlying tissues. The severity of the damage is determined by the duration of exposure, the type of agent delivering the energy, and the temperature to which the skin is exposed [1, 2].

Burn injuries may result from multiple mechanisms, including friction, extreme cold, heat, radiation, chemical agents, or electrical sources. However, most burns occur due to thermal exposure from hot liquids, heated surfaces, or open flames [2].

The inflammatory and stress responses following burn injury are marked by increased circulating concentrations of cytokines, chemokines, and acute-phase proteins, accompanied by a pronounced hypermetabolic state. This metabolic response is largely driven by sustained sympathetic activation, which may extend well beyond the initial acute phase of treatment.

The intensity of the host response is multifactorial and influenced by several variables, including the severity of the burn – reflected by total body surface area (TBSA) involvement and depth of injury – the etiologic mechanism of the burn, and the presence of associated inhalation injury or toxic exposures. Additional contributors include concomitant traumatic injuries and patient-specific factors such as age, preexisting comorbid conditions, substance intoxication, and delays in access to definitive medical care [3, 4].

Immediately following a burn injury, the wound is classically described as comprising three concentric zones. The central zone of coagulation represents the area of maximal and irreversible tissue damage. Surrounding this region is the zone of stasis, also referred to as the ischemic zone, which is characterized by reduced perfusion and cellular injury that remains potentially reversible if timely interventions are implemented. The outermost zone of hyperemia exhibits increased blood flow secondary to inflammatory vasodilation and is typically associated with minimal structural damage. The extent and nature of cellular injury differ across these zones and encompass a continuum of biological responses. These range from early cellular autophagy occurring within the first 24 hours after injury to delayed apoptotic processes emerging approximately 24–48 hours post-burn, as well as reversible injury mediated by oxidative stress [5].

As previously mentioned, immediately after thermal injury, the burn wound can be conceptualized as three concentric zones of tissue damage (see **Figure 1**), as originally described in the classic Jackson model. The central zone of coagulation corresponds to the area of maximal injury, with irreversible protein denaturation and cellular necrosis. Surrounding it lies the zone of stasis (ischemia), characterized by reduced microvascular perfusion and inflammation; importantly, this region is *potentially salvageable* but remains vulnerable to secondary ischemic progression ("burn wound conversion") within the first 24–48 hours. The outer zone of hyperemia represents the most peripheral region, where inflammatory vasodilation increases blood flow, and tissue is generally expected to recover [5].

3. Microvascular disruption and interstitial matrix disruption

An understanding of microvascular fluid balance and transcapillary exchange is essential to explain the profound hemodynamic and tissue changes that occur following burn injury. Under normal physiologic conditions, intravascular volume is

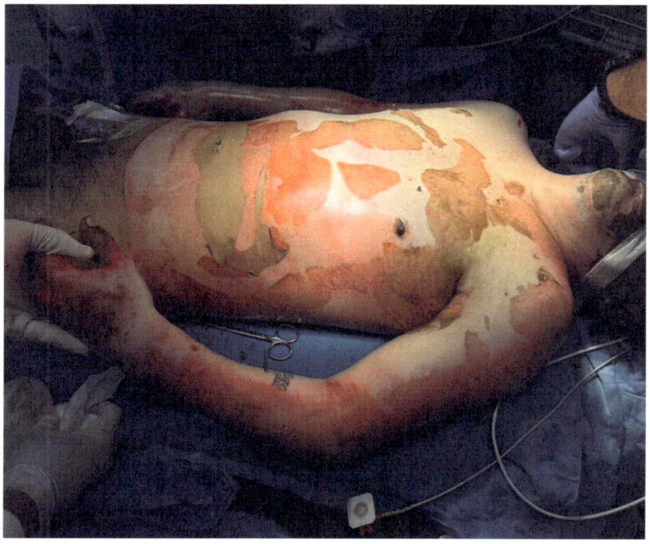

Figure 1.
Clinical image of burn zones.

maintained, and edema formation is limited by the balance of forces described by the Starling equation, which governs net fluid movement across the capillary wall:

$$Q_f = K[(P_{mv} - P_i) - \sigma(\pi_{mv} - \pi_i)]$$

where Q represents the net fluid filtration rate from the intravascular space to the interstitium; Kf is the capillary filtration coefficient determined by capillary surface area and interstitial compliance; Pc and Pi are capillary and interstitial hydrostatic pressures, respectively; σ is the reflection coefficient representing capillary permeability; and πc and πi are plasma and interstitial oncotic pressures. Under physiologic conditions, fluid filtered into the interstitium is efficiently cleared by the lymphatic system, thereby preventing clinically significant edema formation [6].

The structural integrity of the interstitial space is maintained by hyaluronic acid, collagen, and proteoglycans, which exist in a coiled configuration that generates a negative elastic force opposing fluid accumulation.

Following a burn injury, microvascular disruption and extracellular matrix damage result in the loss of this restraining force. As edema develops, tissue compliance increases disproportionately relative to pressure, leading to progressive uncoiling of the interstitial matrix and facilitating further extravasation of fluid into the extravascular space. This process establishes a self-perpetuating cycle of edema formation [6, 7].

4. Hypermetabolism

After a severe burn injury, the systemic metabolic response typically unfolds in two distinct phases. During the first 72–96 hours, an early hypometabolic "ebb" phase predominates, characterized by reduced energy expenditure, decreased intravascular volume, low cardiac output, and inadequate tissue perfusion. This early period is thought to reflect acute cellular constraints on metabolic capacity, including mitochondrial dysfunction and increased endoplasmic reticulum stress.

Patients then transition into a hypermetabolic "flow" phase, which is most pronounced in extensive burns and can persist for prolonged periods – reported up to 36 months after the initial insult. This state is marked by sustained elevations in resting energy expenditure, hyperthermia, peripheral insulin resistance, and profound catabolism. A central driver is persistent neuroendocrine activation, with increased catecholamines, glucocorticoids, glucagon, and dopamine, promoting accelerated glycogenolysis, proteolysis, and lipolysis.

Consequently, there is a rapid loss of skeletal muscle and total body protein, accompanied by an exaggerated acute-phase response. Although some acute-phase mediators (including IGF-1) may exert anabolic signaling, the net balance remains strongly catabolic, contributing to progressive organ dysfunction, including multi-organ failure, and increased mortality risk. Importantly, while comparable stress-metabolic patterns occur in trauma and critical illness, severe burns are distinguished by their magnitude and duration, likely amplified by sustained inflammatory mediator release (e.g., interleukin-1 [IL-1], interleukin-6 [IL-6], tumor necrosis factor [TNF], and other cytokines/chemokines).

More recently, burn-associated "browning" of white adipose tissue has been described, in which inflammation and adrenergic signaling induce a thermogenic phenotype with upregulation of uncoupling protein-1 (UCP1), increasing mitochondrial uncoupling and energy consumption, and further contributing to hypermetabolism and immunometabolic dysregulation [4, 6].

5. Damage-associated molecular patterns/pathogen-associated molecular patterns

Once the key points regarding the hypermetabolic response have been reviewed, it is important to note that burn injuries also exert a profound impact on the immune system. Innate immune cells – including monocytes, macrophages, and neutrophils – are rapidly activated in response to burn trauma. Within hours, endogenous mediators, such as DAMPs, are generated as a consequence of burn-induced tissue injury [4].

Damage-associated molecular patterns, together with their exogenous counterparts known as PAMPs, are recognized by pattern-recognition receptors (PRRs), particularly Toll-like receptors (TLRs) and NOD-like receptors (NLRs). Engagement of TLRs and NLRs triggers downstream inflammatory signaling pathways, culminating in the activation of nuclear factor kappa B (NF-κB), a central transcription factor that promotes the expression and release of pro-inflammatory mediators, including ILs and TNF [4].

6. Multiple organ dysfunction after burn injury

Severe burn injury induces a profound and sustained systemic response that frequently culminates in multiple organ dysfunction syndrome (MODS), a leading cause of late morbidity and mortality in burn patients. Importantly, the pathogenesis of MODS following burns extends beyond hypovolemia or inadequate resuscitation and reflects a complex interaction between inflammatory mediators, cellular injury pathways, metabolic derangements, and neuroendocrine stress responses [8].

7. Cardiovascular dysfunction

A reduction in cardiac output represents one of the earliest manifestations of burn-induced organ dysfunction, occurring despite adequate fluid resuscitation. Experimental and clinical studies have demonstrated that, although fluid therapy improves preload, it does not fully restore left ventricular contractility, even under conditions of maximal preload and preserved coronary blood flow. Animal models with burns exceeding 45% TBSA have shown impaired isovolumetric relaxation, reduced diastolic compliance, and depressed left ventricular contractility, underscoring an intrinsic myocardial dysfunction rather than a purely preload-dependent phenomenon [7].

Biochemical evidence further supports direct myocardial injury. Elevated cardiac troponin I levels have been detected in both animal models and humans following major burns, particularly in patients with burns greater than 20% TBSA, where elevations persist for up to 12 hours after injury. In contrast, troponin elevations are not observed in smaller burns (<10% TBSA), suggesting a threshold-dependent myocardial insult. Temporal analyses indicate that myocardial dysfunction may begin as early as 2 hours post-injury, with partial or complete resolution typically occurring between 48 and 72 hours [8].

Pro-inflammatory cytokines play a central role in mediating this cardiac dysfunction. Elevated serum levels of TNF-α, IL-1β, and IL-6 have consistently been demonstrated in thermally injured patients compared with controls. Administration of TNF-α to healthy volunteers reproduces cardiac changes similar to those observed after burn injury, implicating this cytokine as a key mediator. Experimental studies have further shown that TNF-α blockade improves myocardial contractility in burned animals, reinforcing its pathogenic role. Oxidative stress also contributes significantly; antioxidant therapy with vitamins A, C, E, and zinc has been shown to preserve myocardial contractility, reduce nuclear translocation of nuclear factor-κB, and attenuate cytokine production within cardiomyocytes [9].

Apoptosis has emerged as an additional mechanism of burn-induced myocardial dysfunction. In rat models of 40% TBSA full-thickness burns, increased cardiomyocyte apoptosis – particularly within the subendocardial region – has been observed at 24 hours and persists at 48 hours. The extent of apoptosis correlates closely with left ventricular pressure dysfunction, suggesting that programmed cell death contributes meaningfully to early cardiac failure after burn injury [10].

8. Metabolic, endocrine, and hepatic dysfunction

Beyond the heart, burn injury induces widespread metabolic and endocrine derangements that contribute to MODS. Early after burn injury, significant increases in complement C3, α2-microglobulin, haptoglobin, and C-reactive protein are observed, while levels of prealbumin, transferrin, and apolipoprotein A1 decline markedly, reflecting a hepatic reprioritization toward inflammatory protein synthesis. Large cohort analyses of severely burned children (TBSA > 30%) have demonstrated immediate and sustained hypermetabolism, with resting energy expenditure increasing to approximately 130% of predicted values shortly after injury. This hypermetabolic state is accompanied by profound alterations in acute-phase reactants and constitutively produced hepatic proteins [11].

The inflammatory cytokine response is both broad and intense. Marked elevations have been documented in a wide array of mediators, including IL-2, IL-4, IL-6, IL-8, IL-10, IL-17, TNF-α, IL-1β, interferon-γ, granulocyte–macrophage colony-stimulating factor, monocyte chemotactic protein-1, and macrophage inflammatory proteins. Although the precise role of each cytokine remains incompletely defined, their collective impact underscores the magnitude and persistence of systemic inflammation following burn trauma. Hepatic enlargement further reflects this response, with liver size increasing to approximately 180% of predicted values at one week and up to 220% by two weeks post-burn, indicating sustained organ adaptation and stress.

Endocrine changes are similarly extensive. Hyperglycemia and hyperinsulinemia develop within the first day after injury, indicative of acute insulin resistance. Concurrently, insulin-like growth factor-1, thyroxine, and parathyroid hormone levels decrease, whereas cortisol levels in serum and urine rise significantly. These alterations illustrate the catabolic and stress-dominated hormonal milieu characteristic of severe burns [11].

9. Renal and splanchnic dysfunction

Given the early reduction in cardiac output, alterations in regional blood flow have been extensively investigated. Experimental studies assessing radiotracer uptake after moderate burns have demonstrated reduced renal perfusion within minutes of injury, while hepatic and intestinal blood flow appear relatively preserved. These findings suggest that hepatic dysfunction after burns is not primarily ischemic in origin, but rather mediated by inflammatory and metabolic mechanisms.

Acute renal failure (ARF) remains a serious complication of burn injury, with reported incidences ranging from approximately 5% to nearly 30%, depending on

	Key mediators/features	Functional consequence	Downstream outcome
Burn injury	Tissue damage (thermal injury)	Triggers the release of danger and microbial signals	Initiates systemic pathways
DAMPs and PAMPs released	DAMPs: HMGB1, mitochondrial DNA, dsRNA; PAMPs: LPS, peptidoglycans	Activates innate immune sensing and amplifies inflammation	Drives vascular leak, immune dysregulation, and metabolic changes
Hypovolemic shock and vascular leak	Capillary leak and intravascular fluid loss	Decreased effective circulating volume; fluid shifts to interstitium	Tissue edema, tissue injury, increased risk of bacterial infection, increased burn depth, and severity
Immune and inflammatory response (global)	Systemic inflammatory activation with concurrent immune dysfunction	Dysregulated host defense (hyperinflammation + immunoparalysis)	Leads to immunosuppression and impaired bacterial clearance
Monocyte (within immune response)	Increased IL-6, IL-10, TNF, PGE_2; decreased Class II MHC expression; decreased antigen presentation	Reduced adaptive immune priming	Immunosuppression
T cells (within immune response)	Increased IL-4 and IL-10; decreased IL-2 and IFNγ; decreased proliferation	Impaired cell-mediated immunity	Immunosuppression
Macrophage + neutrophil (within immune response)	Decreased phagocytosis; decreased bactericidal activity	Ineffective bacterial killing	Bacterial multiplication
Metabolic changes	Catabolism, insulin resistance, muscle protein degradation, lipolysis	Sustained stress response and substrate mobilization	Hypermetabolism
Intermediate states	Immunosuppression + bacterial multiplication + hypermetabolism	Host becomes vulnerable to infection and systemic dysregulation	SIRS and/or sepsis
Systemic outcome	Escalating systemic inflammation and infection	Organ dysfunction progression	Multiple organ failure ultimately progresses to death

Table 1.
Pathways in sepsis and subsequent multiorgan dysfunction after burn injury.

definitions and patient populations. The development of ARF is associated with dramatically increased mortality, historically approaching 100%, though improvements in resuscitation strategies have reduced mortality to approximately 50–60%. Importantly, more recent studies indicate that early ARF is not necessarily related to resuscitation volume or urine output but rather correlates with the severity of metabolic acidosis and base deficit within the first 24 hours after injury. Elevated base deficit and serum lactate levels appear to reflect the magnitude of the systemic inflammatory response, linking renal dysfunction more closely to global inflammatory burden than to isolated renal hypoperfusion [12–14].

10. Integrative perspective

Collectively, these findings highlight that MODS after burn injury arises from a highly integrated and interdependent systemic response, rather than from isolated organ-specific insults. Cardiovascular depression, metabolic and endocrine dysregulation, hepatic acute-phase responses, and renal dysfunction are all interconnected through inflammatory mediators, oxidative stress, and cellular injury pathways(see **Table 1.**). While advances in supportive care have improved survival, these same data underscore the challenge of therapeutic intervention: Targeting a single mediator or pathway may yield both beneficial and detrimental downstream effects. Future progress in reducing burn-related MODS will likely depend on strategies that modulate the global inflammatory and metabolic response, rather than focusing solely on individual organ dysfunction.

Acknowledgments

The authors acknowledge using ChatGPT for language editing in the chapter.

Conflict of Interest

The authors declare no conflicts of interest.

Author details

Alhan Fernando
Castillo Valencia, Autonomous University of Guadalajara, Guadalajara, Mexico

*Address all correspondence to: alhancastillo@hotmail.com

References

[1] Kaddoura I, Abu-Sittah G, Ibrahim A, Karamanoukian R, Papazian N. Burn injury: Review of pathophysiology and therapeutic modalities in major burns. Ann Burns Fire Disasters. 2017;**30**(2):95–102

[2] Lund T, Onarheim H, Reed RK. Pathogenesis of edema formation in burn injuries. World Journal of Surgery. 1992;**16**(1):2–9

[3] Żwierełło W, Piorun K, Skórka-Majewicz M, Maruszewska A, Antoniewski J, Gutowska I. Burns: Classification, Pathophysiology, and Treatment: A Review. International Journal of Molecular Sciences. 2023;**24** 1–17. DOI: 10.3390/ ijms24043749

[4] Jeschke MG, van Baar ME, Choudhry MA, Chung KK, Gibran NS, Logsetty S. Burn injury. Nature Reviews Disease Primers. 2020;**6**(1):11

[5] Jeschke MG, Chinkes DL, Finnerty CC, Kulp G, Suman OE, Norbury WB, et al. Pathophysiologic response to severe burn injury. Annals of Surgery. 2008;**248**(3):387–401. DOI: 10.1097/ SLA.0b013e3181856241

[6] Rae L, Fidler P, Gibran N. The Physiologic Basis of Burn Shock and the Need for Aggressive Fluid Resuscitation. Critical Care Clinics. 2016;**32**:491–505. DOI: 10.1016/j.ccc.2016.06.001

[7] Demling RH. The burn edema process: Current concepts. Journal of Burn Care and Rehabilitation. 2005;**26** (3):207–227

[8] Evans EI, Purnell OJ, Robinett PW, Batchelor A, Martin M. Fluid and electrolyte requirements in severe burns. Annals of Surgery. 1952;**135**(6): 804–815. DOI: 10.1097/00000658-195 206000-00006

[9] Adams HR, Baxter CR, Izenberg SD. Decreased contractility and compliance of the left ventricle as complications of thermal trauma. American Heart Journal. 1984;**108**(6):1477–1487

[10] Murphy JT, Horton JW, Purdue GF, Hunt JL. Evaluation of troponin-I as an indicator of cardiac dysfunction after thermal injury. Journal of Trauma. 1998;**45**(4): 700–707

[11] Sweeney TE, Shidham A, Wong HR, Khatri P.A comprehensive time-course-based multicohort analysis of sepsis and sterile inflammation reveals a robust diagnostic gene set. Science Translational Medicine. 2015;**7** (287). DOI: 10.1126/scitranslmed. aaa5993

[12] Carlson DL, Horton JW. Cardiac molecular signaling after burn trauma. Journal of Burn Care and Research. 2006;**27**(5):669–675

[13] Jeschke MG. The Hepatic Response to Thermal Injury: Is the Liver Important for Postburn Outcomes? Molecular Medicine. 2009;**15**(9):337–351

[14] Mustonen KM, Vuola J. Acute renal failure in intensive care burn patients (ARF in burn patients). Journal of Burn Care and Research. 2008;**29**(1):227–237

Chapter 2

Pathophysiology-Driven Treatment Strategies in Burn Injury

Ovunc Akdemir

Abstract

Burn injury is a dynamic form of trauma in which an initial cutaneous insult triggers a time-dependent cascade of microvascular failure, inflammation, immune dysregulation, and sustained hypermetabolism. These processes govern burn wound progression, infection risk, quality of healing, and the probability of hypertrophic scarring and contracture. A pathophysiology-driven approach allows clinicians to match treatment intensity and timing to biologic behavior rather than surface appearance alone. This chapter synthesizes key mechanisms – zones of injury, endothelial and microcirculatory dysfunction, oxidative stress, cytokine signaling, and fibroproliferative remodeling – and links them to practical decision-making in acute care and reconstruction. We highlight how controlled resuscitation, early excision when indicated, targeted wound-bed preparation, negative pressure wound therapy, and contemporary cell-based epidermal regeneration can be integrated into a reconstructive strategy focused on function, esthetics, and long-term quality of life. Special considerations for chemical and electrical injuries and the elderly burn patient are discussed, along with emerging directions in biologic modulation and regenerative medicine.

Keywords: burn injury, pathophysiology, microcirculation, hypermetabolism, infection, negative pressure wound therapy, cell-based therapy, scar, contracture, reconstruction

1. Introduction

Burn injury represents a unique form of trauma in which localized tissue destruction may rapidly evolve into a complex, multisystem disorder [1–5]. Unlike conventional wounds, burns initiate a cascade of microvascular, inflammatory, metabolic, and immunologic events that profoundly influence both acute survival and long-term functional outcomes. Despite advances in resuscitation and critical care, morbidity related to impaired wound healing, infection, contracture, and pathologic scarring remains substantial [3, 6–10].

Traditional burn management has relied on the extent and apparent depth of injury as the primary determinants of treatment strategy [1, 3]. Although these parameters are clinically indispensable, they do not fully reflect the dynamic biologic processes that govern tissue viability, wound progression, and reparative capacity [2, 4]. Therapeutic decisions based solely on surface appearance risk overlooking microcirculatory failure, immune dysregulation, and molecular signaling abnormalities that directly influence outcomes [4, 9].

From a plastic and reconstructive surgery perspective, effective burn care extends beyond wound closure. A rational strategy requires understanding why tissue fails, how healing becomes dysregulated, and when reconstruction should be biologically – rather than purely temporally – driven [11]. The timing of surgical intervention, selection of wound coverage techniques, use of adjunctive therapies such as negative pressure wound therapy (NPWT) or cell-based treatments, and prevention of contracture and fibrosis are all influenced by the evolving pathophysiology of burn injury [12, 13].

This chapter adopts a mechanism-oriented framework for burn management, integrating fundamental cellular and molecular events with contemporary clinical practice [6, 11, 14]. The objective is to provide a surgeon-oriented approach, aligning treatment strategies with the biologic behavior of different burn types and severities, translating pathophysiologic principles into practical decisions across the continuum of care [3, 4, 15].

2. Pathophysiology of burn injury

2.1 Local tissue response and the zones of burn injury

The immediate consequence of burn injury is the direct damage to the skin and underlying tissues through thermal, chemical, or electrical mechanisms [3, 16–20]. The classical description of burn wounds as comprising three concentric zones – coagulation, stasis, and hyperemia – remains clinically relevant [1, 2].

The zone of coagulation represents irreversible necrosis caused by protein denaturation, membrane disruption, and loss of cellular homeostasis [1, 2]. Surrounding this is the zone of stasis, a metabolically compromised but potentially viable region characterized by impaired perfusion, endothelial injury, and increased capillary permeability [2, 5]. The outermost zone of hyperemia exhibits vasodilation and increased blood flow, and it typically recovers in the absence of secondary insults [1, 2].

Burn wound progression reflects the biologic vulnerability of the zone of stasis. Microvascular thrombosis, interstitial edema, and mediator-driven endothelial dysfunction may convert salvageable tissue into full-thickness necrosis over hours to days [5, 9, 21–23]. Clinically, this supports early strategies that preserve microcirculation and limit secondary tissue loss, including controlled resuscitation, avoidance of unnecessary desiccation or pressure, timely debridement when indicated, and rational adjunctive therapies [3, 15] (**Figure 1**, **Table 1**).

This figure illustrates the fundamental pathophysiologic mechanisms underlying thermal, chemical, and electrical burn injuries in relation to tissue depth. The classical zones of burn injury – coagulation, stasis, and hyperemia – highlight gradients of tissue viability and microcirculatory compromise. Thermal burns result in protein denaturation and coagulative necrosis, chemical burns cause ongoing tissue destruction depending on the agent, and electrical burns produce deep tissue

DOI: http://dx.doi.org/10.5772/intechopen.1014625

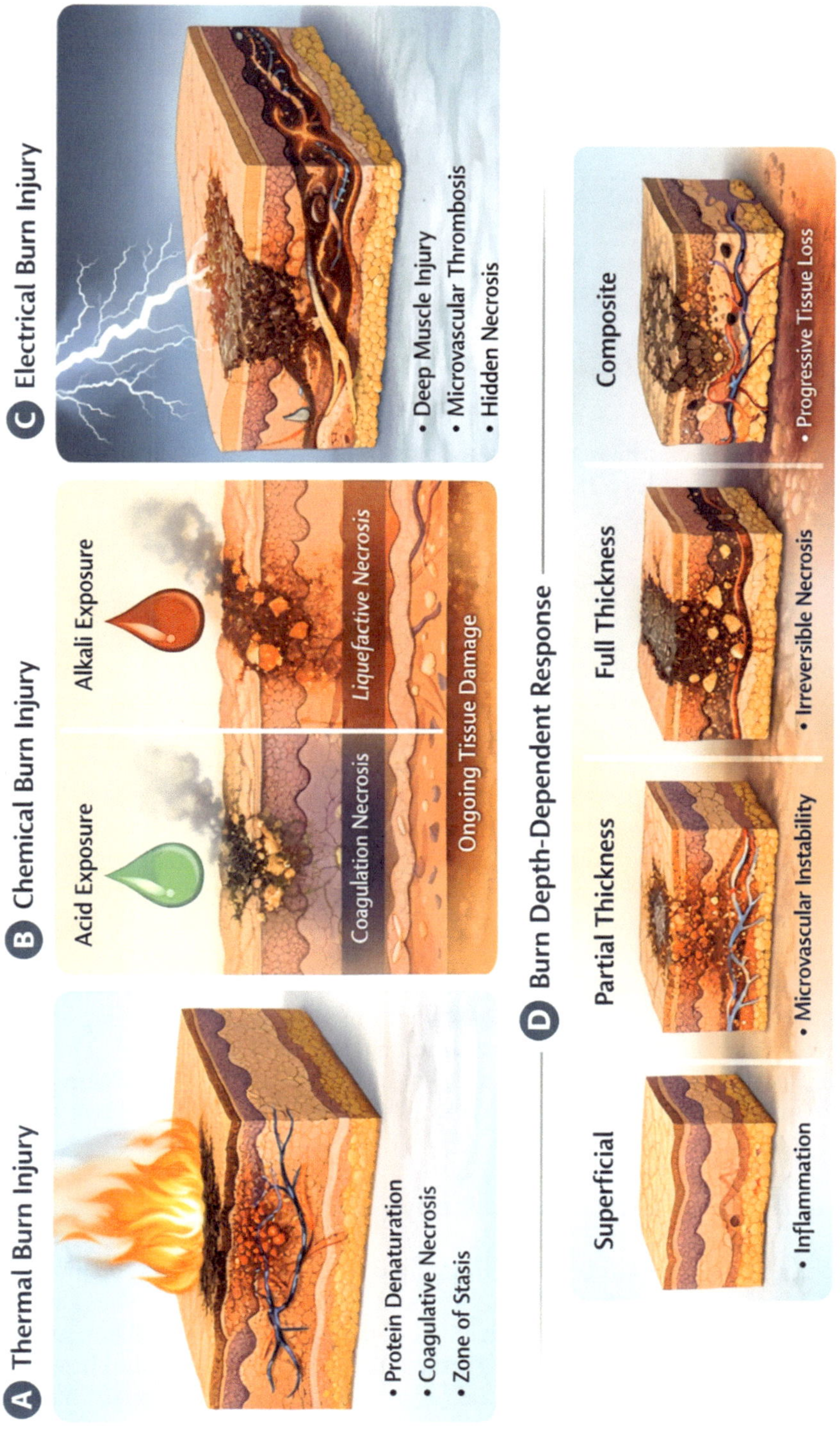

Figure 1.
Pathophysiology of burn injury according to burn type and depth.

Burn depth/type	Dominant pathophysiology	Key biologic risk	Treatment strategy
Superficial (thermal)	Inflammation	Barrier loss	Nonoperative management
Partial thickness (thermal)	Microcirculatory failure	Wound conversion	NPWT, selective excision
Full thickness (thermal)	Irreversible necrosis	Infection, fibrosis	Early excision and grafting or flap surgery
Electrical	Microthrombosis, ischemia	Deep necrosis	Staged debridement, flap reconstruction
Chemical	Ongoing tissue injury	Progressive damage	Immediate irrigation, delayed reconstruction

Table 1.
Pathophysiology-based treatment alignment in burn injury.

injury with limited cutaneous findings. The figure emphasizes burn wound progression and provides a framework for pathophysiology-driven treatment strategies.

2.2 Microcirculatory dysfunction and endothelial injury

Microvascular failure is a central event in burn pathophysiology [2, 5, 9]. Endothelial cells sustain direct injury from the insult and indirect injury mediated by cytokines, complement activation, and oxidative stress [9, 22–28]. Increased vascular permeability causes plasma extravasation and interstitial edema, which elevates tissue pressure and compromises capillary blood flow [5, 9].

As edema progresses, diffusion distances increase, and local oxygen delivery worsens. Concurrent hemoconcentration and platelet activation promote microthrombus formation, further impairing perfusion in vulnerable tissue [2, 9, 29]. These changes can be more pronounced in deep burns and in injuries with extensive subdermal damage – particularly electrical and chemical burns – where skin findings may underestimate microvascular compromise [18–20].

From a treatment standpoint, the goal is to restore and maintain adequate perfusion with the smallest effective resuscitation volume, limit ongoing edema, and decompress threatened compartments when necessary [3, 15, 30–33]. These principles explain why overresuscitation can paradoxically worsen tissue viability and why escharotomy is often as much a physiologic intervention as it is a technical procedure.

2.3 Inflammatory cascade and immune dysregulation

Burn injury triggers a robust inflammatory response initiated by damage-associated molecular patterns released from necrotic tissue [4, 9]. These signals activate resident immune cells and drive systemic release of proinflammatory mediators, including tumor necrosis factor-alpha, interleukin-1β, and interleukin-6 [4, 9, 34–38]. Inflammation is essential for debris clearance and repair initiation; however, excessive or prolonged activation contributes to endothelial dysfunction, capillary leak, and delayed epithelialization [9, 38–43].

Systemically, major burns may produce a biphasic immune phenotype: an early hyperinflammatory state followed by functional immunosuppression [4, 17, 44–47]. Neutrophil dysfunction and dysregulated lymphocyte responses increase susceptibility to infection and sepsis [8, 17, 47]. These immune changes are clinically meaningful for reconstruction because infection risk and graft reliability are tied to the inflammatory and immunologic milieu.

2.4 Oxidative stress and redox signaling

Oxidative stress is a key driver of early tissue injury and a regulator of subsequent healing. Reactive oxygen species and reactive nitrogen species can amplify endothelial damage, promote lipid peroxidation, and impair mitochondrial function, leading to apoptosis or necrosis in vulnerable cells [45].

At the same time, controlled redox signaling is not purely deleterious; physiologic levels of reactive species participate in antimicrobial defense and act as second messengers in wound repair [45]. Severe burns can shift this balance toward persistent oxidative injury, contributing to delayed epithelialization and exaggerated fibroproliferation. Clinically, reducing the inflammatory burden (timely debridement, infection control) and optimizing perfusion indirectly modulate redox stress.

2.5 Molecular and cellular mediators of tissue injury and repair

Burn injury disrupts coordinated interactions among keratinocytes, fibroblasts, endothelial cells, and immune cells – interactions central to reepithelialization and matrix remodeling [42–44]. Key signaling axes include growth factor pathways that regulate migration, proliferation, angiogenesis, and extracellular matrix deposition.

Vascular endothelial growth factor supports angiogenesis and vascular remodeling but may also contribute to increased permeability early on [22]. Transforming growth factor-beta signaling promotes fibroblast activation and collagen deposition, linking early inflammation to later fibrosis and hypertrophic scar formation [10, 24, 25, 48, 49]. Platelet-derived growth factor supports fibroblast chemotaxis and matrix synthesis – beneficial for closure but potentially pathologic when persistent [44].

These mechanisms justify a strategy focused on timely closure (to shorten inflammatory exposure), tension control (to reduce profibrotic signaling), and the selective use of dermal substitutes or biologic adjuncts when the wound bed biology is suboptimal [15, 26, 27].

2.6 Hypermetabolic response and systemic catabolism

Major burns induce a sustained hypermetabolic state mediated by catecholamines, cortisol, and inflammatory cytokines [9, 30]. Resting energy expenditure increases, accompanied by protein catabolism, insulin resistance, and loss of lean body mass [9, 30].

This systemic environment impairs wound healing by limiting substrate availability for collagen synthesis and angiogenesis, and by reducing immune competence [30]. For reconstructive surgeons, this supports early nutritional optimization and careful staging to match reconstructive complexity to the patient's physiology [30].

2.7 Aberrant healing, fibrosis, and contracture formation

Pathologic scarring remains a major long-term burden after burn injury. Prolonged inflammation, delayed epithelialization, and mechanical tension promote excessive fibroblast activity and abnormal collagen architecture, resulting in hypertrophic scarring and contracture formation [10, 23–25].

Following a burn injury, wound healing is initiated through a highly coordinated sequence of cellular migration and differentiation events. During the early inflammatory phase, neutrophils migrate into the wound bed to clear necrotic debris and microbial contaminants, followed by macrophages that orchestrate subsequent repair through cytokine and growth factor release. As inflammation subsides, keratinocytes migrate from the wound edges and residual epidermal appendages to restore epithelial continuity, while fibroblasts migrate into the provisional extracellular matrix to synthesize collagen and provide structural support [38, 43].

Under physiologic conditions, fibroblast activity is tightly regulated and gradually diminishes as reepithelialization and tissue remodeling progress. However, in burn wounds characterized by prolonged inflammation, delayed closure, or excessive mechanical tension, fibroblasts differentiate into contractile myofibroblasts. These cells generate sustained contractile forces and deposit densely packed collagen fibers, leading to progressive tissue shortening and scar contracture formation. Persistent myofibroblast activation and failure of normal apoptotic resolution represent key biologic mechanisms underlying hypertrophic scarring and functional impairment after burn injury [49].

This cellular continuum – from inflammatory cell infiltration to aberrant fibroblast-driven contraction – highlights that burn contracture is not merely a mechanical sequela but the consequence of dysregulated wound biology, reinforcing the need for early wound modulation and timely reconstructive intervention [23, 38, 40–45, 49] (**Figure 2**)

This figure demonstrates the sequential cellular events involved in burn wound healing and the mechanisms leading to scar contracture formation.

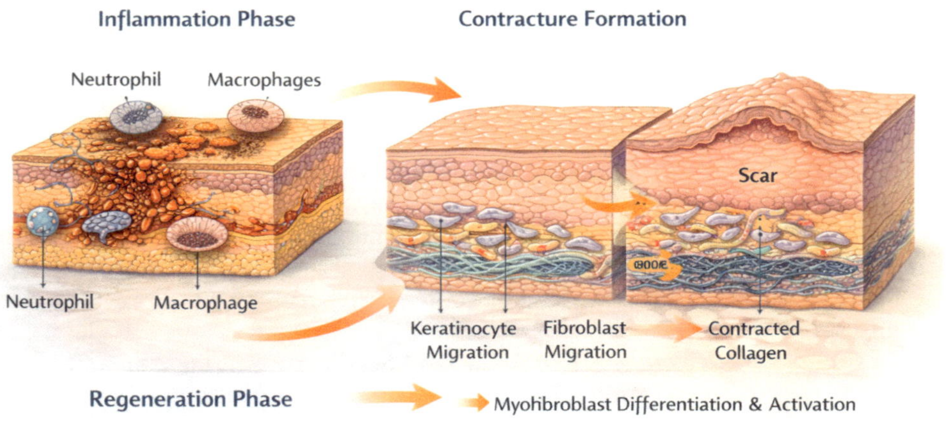

Figure 2.
Cellular migration and mechanisms of contracture formation during burn wound healing.

Neutrophils and macrophages initiate debris clearance and cytokine signaling. Keratinocyte migration enables reepithelialization, while fibroblast activity supports extracellular matrix deposition. Under conditions of prolonged inflammation, delayed wound closure, or excessive mechanical tension, fibroblasts differentiate into myofibroblasts, resulting in sustained contraction, excessive collagen deposition, and hypertrophic scar formation.

Contracture prevention begins during acute care through strategies that shorten the time to closure, optimize the wound environment, and reduce prolonged inflammation and tension. International scar management principles emphasize early closure and structured rehabilitation to limit contracture risk [41].

3. Pathophysiology-driven acute and early burn management

3.1 Resuscitation principles guided by microcirculation

Early burn management aims not only to stabilize the patient but also to preserve tissue biology [3, 15]. Excessive resuscitation can worsen interstitial edema and impair microcirculation, while inadequate resuscitation perpetuates ischemia [5, 9]. Resuscitation should be titrated to physiologic endpoints, balancing perfusion with the avoidance of unnecessary edema [3, 15] (**Table 2**).

3.2 Early excision and wound bed optimization

Necrotic tissue sustains inflammation and bacterial growth and creates a hostile wound bed. Early excision, when feasible, reduces the mediator burden and accelerates conversion to a wound environment more permissive for angiogenesis and epithelialization [15]. In selected patients, early excision and grafting can reduce complications and improve outcomes [15, 50].

Dermal substitutes and biomaterials may improve matrix architecture and decrease contraction in selected settings, particularly when native dermis is deficient [26, 27].

3.3 Infection control as a pathophysiologic intervention

Burn wounds are uniquely susceptible to infection due to the loss of barrier function, immune dysregulation, and devitalized tissue [8, 17]. Infection can drive

Burn type	Depth progression	Microvascular injury	Demarcation	Reconstructive implication
Thermal	Predictable	Moderate	Early	Early grafting
Chemical (acid)	Coagulative	Moderate	Variable	Delayed planning
Chemical (alkali)	Liquefactive	Severe	Late	Staged excision
Electrical	Deep, occult	Severe	Very late	Flap reconstruction mandatory

Table 2.
Comparative pathophysiology of burn types.

further tissue loss by amplifying inflammation and worsening microcirculatory dysfunction; therefore, infection control must be integrated with surgical planning [8, 17].

3.4 NPWT

NPWT modulates the wound microenvironment by reducing edema, improving perfusion, and supporting granulation tissue formation [12, 13]. It can stabilize biologically unstable wounds and serve as a bridge to definitive closure, particularly in complex wounds or challenging anatomical regions [12, 13].

4. Reconstructive strategies from a plastic surgeon's perspective

4.1 Timing reconstruction by biology

In burn reconstruction, timing is dictated by biologic readiness rather than chronology [11, 15, 37]. Reconstruction is optimally undertaken when inflammation is controlled, perfusion is adequate, and systemic conditions support regeneration [15].

4.2 Skin grafting and dermal substitutes

Skin grafting remains central to burn reconstruction, but outcomes depend on vascularity, bacterial burden, and systemic physiology [15, 50]. Dermal substitutes can improve matrix organization and may mitigate contraction in selected cases [26, 27].

4.3 Tissue expansion and skin stretching

Tissue expansion replaces scarred tissue with adjacent, color- and texture-matched skin while minimizing donor morbidity [33]. Controlled skin stretching can facilitate closure in scar excision procedures and reduce the need for multistage reconstruction [34] (**Figure 3**).

This figure demonstrates the staged reconstruction of a nine-year-old patient with severe cervico-axillary contractures following a thermal burn injury.

(a and b) Preoperative views showing extensive contractures with limited neck extension and restricted shoulder abduction. (c) Tissue expansion and contracture release with Z-plasty reconstruction. (d) Twelve-month follow-up demonstrating restored cervical extension. (e–g) Sustained improvement in shoulder mobility with the ability to elevate both upper extremities.

This case highlights the effectiveness of tissue expansion and local flap reconstruction in pediatric burn contracture management.

4.4 Cell-based epidermal regeneration

Cultured epithelial autograft and autologous epidermal cell suspension systems address the loss of epidermal reservoirs and can accelerate epithelialization [31, 32]. These approaches are used as biologic adjuncts, particularly in cases where rapid epithelialization may improve scar quality [31, 32]. Autologous epidermal cell

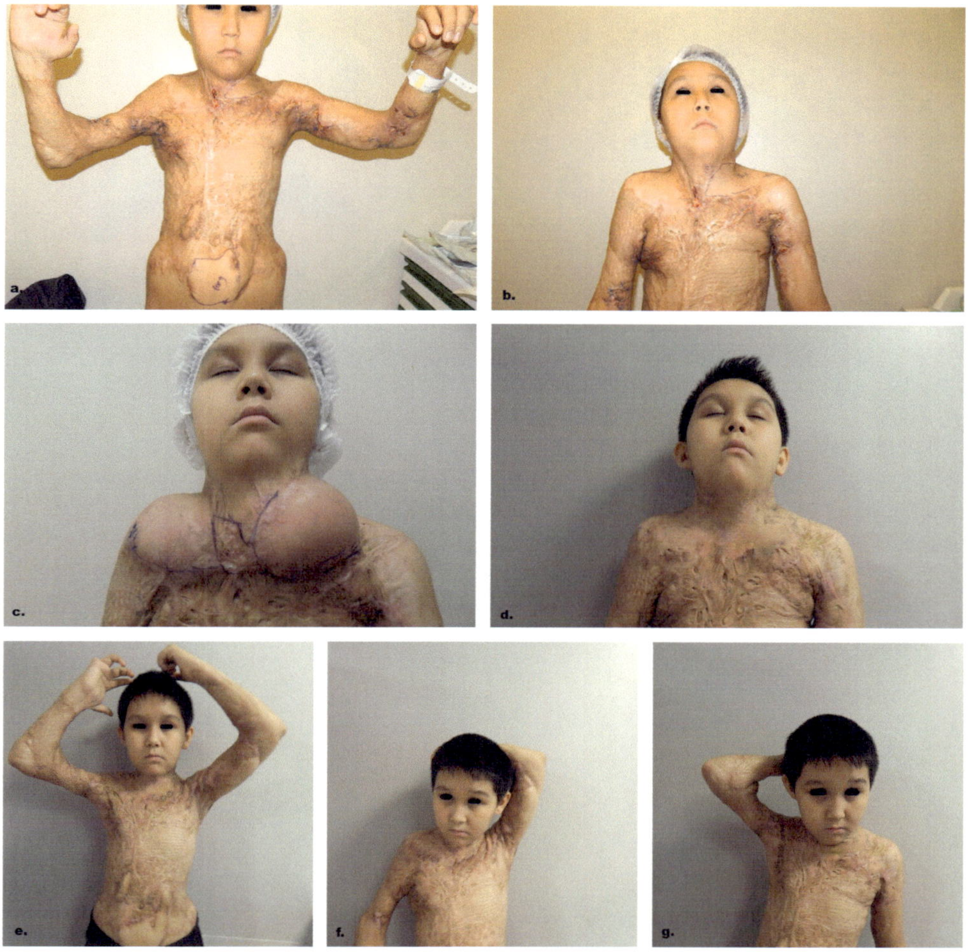

Figure 3.
Contracture-oriented reconstruction following severe pediatric thermal burn injury.

suspension techniques enable the harvesting of a small split-thickness skin sample, followed by enzymatic dissociation into keratinocytes and other epidermal cells, which are subsequently applied to the burn wound as a spray-on micrograft. Commercially available systems, such as ReCell®, have facilitated the standardized clinical application of this approach (**Figure 4**).

This figure illustrates the staged management of a 52-year-old patient with combined high-voltage electrical and thermal burns.

(a) Initial presentation with extensive facial and upper extremity involvement. (b) Dermabrasion for wound bed modulation. (c) Application of biologic therapy to enhance wound healing. (d) Preparation of autologous epidermal cell suspension (ReCell®). (e) Application of biologic therapy to the electrically injured hand. (f and g) Twelve-month follow-up demonstrating satisfactory healing, functional recovery, and acceptable scar quality.

This case demonstrates the integration of biologic adjuncts with reconstructive principles in complex burn management.

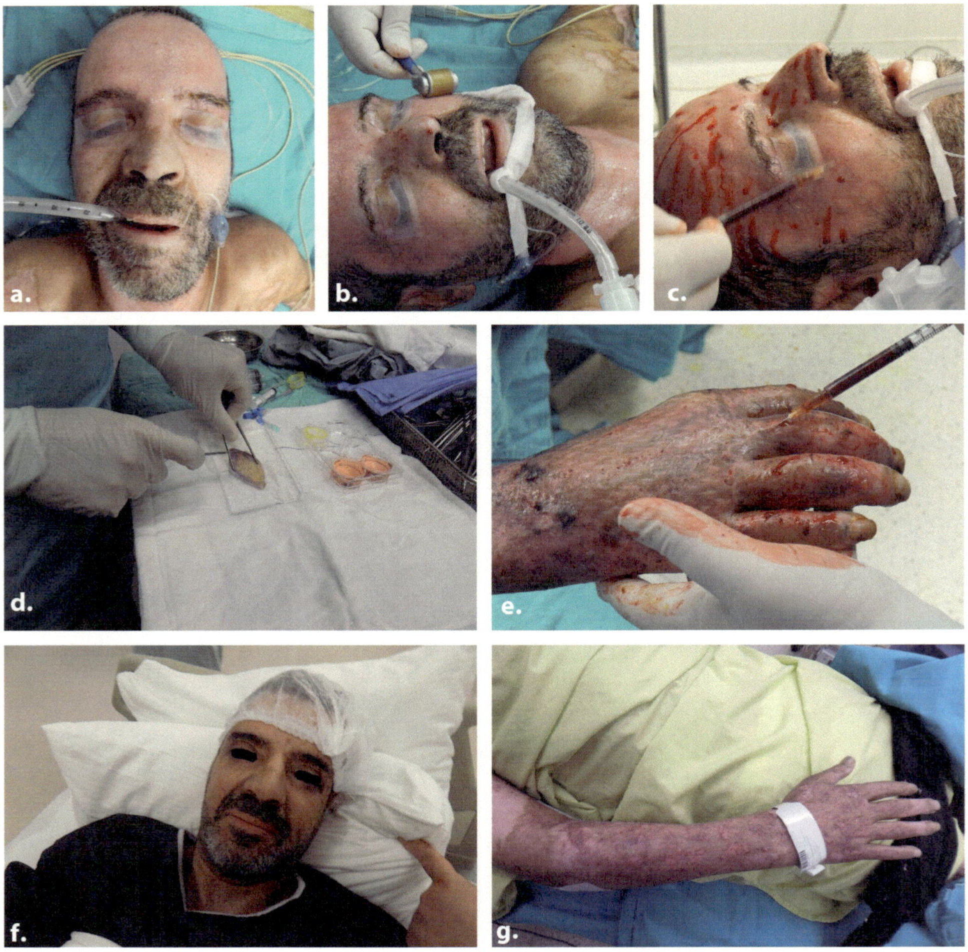

Figure 4.
Multimodal pathophysiology-driven reconstruction in a combined electrical and thermal burn injury.

4.5 Free flap reconstruction

Deep burns, electrical injuries, and composite tissue loss may require free flap reconstruction for durable coverage and functional salvage [19–21]. When performed within an optimized biologic context, vascularized tissue transfer facilitates secondary procedures and long-term restoration [21, 37].

5. Comparative pathophysiology of burn types and severity-oriented treatment strategies

Burn injuries differ fundamentally in biologic behavior depending on etiology and depth, necessitating tailored treatment strategies [18–20].

5.1 Thermal burns

Thermal burns cause protein denaturation and coagulative necrosis. Injury progression occurs primarily through microcirculatory compromise within the zone of stasis [1, 2, 5]. Deep partial- and full-thickness burns often require excision and definitive closure [15, 50].

5.2 Chemical burns

Chemical burns are characterized by ongoing tissue destruction until the offending agent is neutralized. Immediate decontamination is a biologic imperative, and staged assessment is often necessary [18].

5.3 Electrical burns

Electrical burns produce disproportionate deep tissue injury with unreliable cutaneous indicators. Microvascular thrombosis, progressive muscle necrosis, and delayed demarcation are characteristic [19, 20]. Staged debridement and vascularized reconstruction are often required [19–21, 37] (**Table 3**).

5.4 Severity-based alignment

Severity-based alignment follows biologic behavior rather than appearance or chronology [2, 3, 15]. Partial-thickness burns benefit from wound modulation and

Mediator/pathway	Direction of change	Primary biologic effect	Clinical implication
TNF-α	↑ Increased	Endothelial activation, apoptosis	Capillary leak, tissue edema
IL-1β	↑ Increased	Amplified inflammation	Delayed epithelialization
IL-6	↑ Increased	Systemic inflammatory response	Hypermetabolism
Reactive oxygen species	↑ Increased	Oxidative cell injury	Burn wound progression
Nitric oxide	Dysregulated	Vasodilation, cytotoxicity	Microcirculatory instability
VEGF	↑ Increased	Angiogenesis, permeability	Early edema, late neovascularization
TGF-β	↑ Increased	Fibroblast activation	Hypertrophic scarring, contracture
PDGF	↑ Increased	Fibroblast migration	Matrix deposition
MMPs	↑ Increased	ECM degradation	Unstable wound bed
Keratinocyte stem cell pool	↓ Decreased	Impaired reepithelialization	Need for cell-based therapy
Endothelial glycocalyx	↓ Degraded	Barrier dysfunction	Plasma leakage, edema
Catecholamines/ cortisol	↑ Increased	Hypermetabolism	Muscle wasting, delayed healing

Table 3.
Key molecular and cellular mediators altered after burn injury and their clinical relevance.

selective excision [5, 15, 38], while full-thickness burns require early excision and definitive coverage [15, 50]. From a reconstructive perspective, PRP and stem cell-based therapies should not be viewed as standalone solutions but rather as potential biologic adjuncts within a pathophysiology-driven treatment strategy. In our clinical approach, definitive wound closure, control of infection, and optimization of perfusion remain fundamental prerequisites. Biologic therapies may find their greatest value in selected scenarios – such as biologically compromised wound beds, delayed healing, or high-risk scarring – where modulation of the local microenvironment could enhance the effectiveness of established surgical techniques. Future integration of these modalities will depend on clearer indications, standardized protocols, and robust clinical evidence rather than empirical or routine use [42–45]. Based on clinical experience, it should be emphasized that when extensive tissue loss is not present, maintaining an optimal wound environment – particularly adequate moisture control and effective infection prevention – allows the burn wound to progress through intrinsic anabolic processes. Under these conditions, fibroblast migration, increased vascular endothelial growth factor expression, neovascularization, and subsequent reepithelialization can lead to satisfactory skin regeneration. However, in the presence of large or composite defects exceeding the intrinsic regenerative capacity of the tissue, reconstructive intervention becomes mandatory, and from a plastic surgeon's perspective, vascularized tissue transfer to the affected area is required to restore form and function.

6. Special considerations and future directions

Elderly burn patients exhibit reduced physiologic reserve and diminished regenerative capacity, requiring individualized strategies [29]. Prevention and systems-level planning remain important determinants of outcomes at the population level [46]. Emerging approaches in regenerative medicine and biologic modulation are promising but must be applied within a sound pathophysiologic framework [22, 42–45] (**Table 4**).

7. Author perspective: Clinical insights from two decades of burn and reconstructive surgery

Over more than two decades of clinical practice in plastic, reconstructive, and burn surgery, I have learned that successful burn management requires a careful

Wound biology	Systemic status	Preferred reconstruction
Low inflammation	Stable	Split-thickness skin graft
Dermal loss	Stable	Dermal substitute
High contracture risk	Stable	Tissue expansion/skin stretching
Composite defect	Optimized	Free flap reconstruction
Poor wound biology	Unstable	Delay with NPWT

Table 4.
Reconstructive options according to biologic readiness.

balance between systemic stabilization, functional reconstruction, and long-term esthetic rehabilitation. In the early phase of treatment, the primary goal is to support the body's own healing capacity while preventing systemic deterioration. In daily clinical practice, this period also requires meticulous wound care in order to reduce fluid loss and maintain a protective wound environment that minimizes the risk of infection. Appropriate burn dressings and careful wound management are essential for stabilizing injured tissues during the acute phase until definitive reconstructive planning becomes possible.

The severity of burn injury is mainly determined by the depth of tissue damage and the total body surface area (TBSA) involved. In clinical experience, full-thickness burns involving more than approximately 10% TBSA – and particularly those exceeding 30% – represent potentially life-threatening conditions that require prompt multidisciplinary management. In these patients, the immediate priority is the preservation of vital organ function, together with maintaining metabolic and hemodynamic stability.

Surgical intervention during the acute phase is usually reserved for specific indications. For example, the development of circumferential eschar may compromise tissue perfusion or increase compartment pressure. In such situations, urgent procedures such as escharotomy or fasciotomy may be necessary to prevent secondary ischemic injury. However, in many burn patients, the reconstructive phase becomes more relevant later in the recovery process, particularly when managing scar formation, contractures, and functional limitations.

One principle that has consistently guided my approach throughout years of practice is that restoring function must always remain the primary objective, while esthetic considerations should be addressed whenever possible. In practical terms, reconstructive planning should aim to achieve the best functional recovery while also preserving or restoring natural anatomical contours. Surgical planning must, therefore, be individualized according to tissue characteristics, anatomical location, and the functional requirements of the affected region. The choice of reconstructive technique – including skin grafts, local flaps, regional flaps, or more complex reconstructive procedures – should always be tailored to the specific needs of each defect, with the goal of protecting vital structures while maintaining acceptable esthetic outcomes.

In my clinical experience, the most successful results are achieved when reconstruction is not guided solely by the need to close a defect but by a broader understanding of tissue biology, functional restoration, and long-term scar behavior.

Another important observation from long-term clinical practice is the dynamic nature of burn wound progression. Although the initial thermal injury determines the apparent depth of damage, the final extent of tissue necrosis often evolves during the hours and days following the original injury. This progression is closely related to microcirculatory instability, endothelial dysfunction, and inflammatory amplification, which may continue to compromise tissue viability after the initial insult. In clinical practice, this phenomenon is particularly evident in deep dermal burns, where tissues that initially appear viable may later deteriorate due to microvascular thrombosis, persistent edema, and impaired perfusion.

These clinical observations are consistent with experimental studies demonstrating that oxidative stress and ischemia–reperfusion-related mechanisms play a significant role in burn wound evolution. Understanding these biologic processes is essential when determining the appropriate timing of reconstructive procedures, since both premature reconstruction in unstable wound conditions and excessive delays may negatively influence outcomes.

Long-term follow-up of burn patients frequently involves the management of hypertrophic scars and keloids, which represent some of the most common late complications after burn injury. These fibroproliferative conditions may lead not only to esthetic deformities but also to functional impairment, particularly when they occur near joints or other mobile anatomical regions. In clinical practice, the treatment strategy largely depends on the degree of functional limitation and the biologic characteristics of the scar tissue.

When contracture or functional restriction is present, treatment may begin with regenerative approaches aimed at improving tissue quality and reducing excessive fibrosis. In selected cases, regenerative strategies, such as stem-cell-based therapies, may be considered as part of early interventions intended to support tissue remodeling. Depending on the severity of the deformity, reconstruction may subsequently proceed with skin grafting or flap-based techniques to restore function and structural stability.

When the primary concern is esthetic rather than functional, treatment often begins with less invasive approaches, such as intralesional corticosteroid injections, laser therapies, and other minimally invasive scar-modulating treatments designed to reduce fibroproliferative activity and improve scar appearance. If these conservative methods fail to produce satisfactory results, more advanced reconstructive options – including scar excision followed by graft or flap reconstruction – may be necessary.

Looking toward the future, developments in regenerative medicine and reconstructive transplantation are likely to further expand the possibilities for treating severe burn deformities. Vascularized composite allotransplantation has already demonstrated the feasibility of reconstructing complex anatomical structures, such as the face, in carefully selected patients. In addition, ongoing research in tissue engineering may open new avenues for reconstructive surgery. In the future, bioengineered tissues – potentially including xenogeneic or chimeric tissue constructs, in which human-compatible tissues may be generated within controlled biologic platforms – may help overcome the current limitations of donor tissue availability.

Although these approaches remain largely experimental, they represent a promising direction for the future of reconstructive surgery in patients with extensive burn sequelae.

Ultimately, the successful management of burn injuries and their long-term consequences depends heavily on the clinical experience and judgment of the reconstructive surgeon. Burn reconstruction should, therefore, not be viewed merely as a technical procedure, but rather as a biologically guided process that integrates burn pathophysiology, microvascular dynamics, regenerative concepts, and reconstructive surgical principles. From a practical surgical perspective, experience remains one of the most important factors in determining the appropriate timing and technique of reconstruction. By combining surgical expertise with a deeper understanding of tissue biology, it becomes possible to achieve meaningful improvements not only in functional recovery but also in esthetic outcomes and overall patient quality of life.

8. Conclusion

Burn injury is a dynamic and multifaceted pathophysiologic process, extending far beyond the initial cutaneous insult [2–4]. Successful management requires the alignment of resuscitation, wound-bed modulation, and reconstruction with the evolving biologic state of the patient and wound [3, 15]. A pathophysiology-driven approach enables rational treatment selection, minimizes secondary injury, and supports the restoration of function and quality of life [10, 23, 50].

AI tools disclosure

The generative artificial intelligence tool, ChatGPT (OpenAI), was used to assist with English language editing and phrasing refinement. All scientific content, literature selection, interpretation, and final manuscript preparation were performed entirely by the author.

Author details

Ovunc Akdemir
Department of Plastic, Aesthetic and Reconstructive Surgery, Istanbul Aydin University, Istanbul, Turkey

*Address all correspondence to: ovuncakdemir@gmail.com

References

[1] Jackson DM. The diagnosis of the depth of burning. Journal of British Surgery. 1953;**40**(164):588–596. DOI: 10.1002/bjs.18004016413

[2] Arturson G. Pathophysiology of the burn wound and pharmacological treatment. The Rudi Hermans Lecture, 1995. Burns. 1996;**22**(4):255–274. DOI: 10.1016/0305-4179(95)00153-0

[3] Greenhalgh DG. Management of Burns. New England Journal of Medicine. 2019;**380**(24):2349–2359. DOI: 10.1056/NEJMra1807442

[4] Jeschke MG, van Baar ME, Choudhry MA, Chung KK, Gibran NS, Logsetty S. Burn injury. Nature Reviews Disease Primers. 2020;**6**(1):11. DOI: 10.1038/s41572-020-0145-5

[5] Sheridan RL. Burn care: Results of technical and organizational progress. JAMA. 2003;**290**(6):719–722. DOI: 10.1001/jama.290.6.719

[6] Demling RH. The burn edema process: Current concepts. The Journal of Burn Care & Rehabilitation. 2005;**26**(3):207–227

[7] Atiyeh BS, Costagliola M, Hayek SN, Dibo SA. Effect of silver on burn wound infection control and healing: Review of the literature. Burns. 2007;**33**(2):139–148. DOI: 10.1016/j.burns.2006.06.010

[8] Church D, Elsayed S, Reid O, Winston B, Lindsay R. Burn wound infections. Clinical Microbiology Reviews. 2006;**19**(2):403–434. DOI: 10.1128/CMR.19.2.403-434.2006

[9] Jeschke MG, Mlcak RP, Finnerty CC, Norbury WB, Gauglitz GG, Kulp GA, Herndon DN. Burn size determines the inflammatory and hypermetabolic response. Critical Care. 2007;**11**(4):R90. DOI: 10.1186/cc6102

[10] Finnerty CC, Jeschke MG, Branski LK, Barret JP, Dziewulski P, Herndon DN. Hypertrophic scarring: The greatest unmet challenge after burn injury. The Lancet. 2016;**388**(10052):1427–1436. DOI: 10.1016/S0140-6736(16)31406-4

[11] Herndon DN. Total Burn Care. 5th ed. Philadelphia: Elsevier; 2018

[12] Orgill DP, Bayer LR. Negative pressure wound therapy: Past, present and future. International Wound Journal. 2013;**10**(Suppl 1):15–19. DOI: 10.1111/iwj.12170

[13] Morykwas MJ, Argenta LC, Shelton-Brown EI, McGuirt W. Vacuum-assisted closure: A new method for wound control and treatment: Animal studies and basic foundation. Annals of Plastic Surgery. 1997;**38**(6):553–562. DOI: 10.1097/00000637-199706000-00001

[14] Kamolz LP, Kitzinger HB, Karle B, Frey M. The treatment of hand burns. Burns. 2009;**35**(3):327–337. DOI: 10.1016/j.burns.2008.08.004

[15] Gibran NS, Heimbach DM. Current status of burn wound pathophysiology. Clinics in Plastic Surgery. 2000;**27**(1):11–22

[16] Atiyeh BS, Ioannovich J, Al-Amm CA, El-Musa KA. Management of acute and chronic open wounds: The importance of moist environment in

optimal wound healing. Current Pharmaceutical Biotechnology. 2002;**3**(3):179–195. DOI: 10.2174/1389201023378283

[17] Brusselaers N, Monstrey S, Snoeij T, Vandijck D, Lizy C, Hoste E, Lauwaert S, Colpaert K, Vandekerckhove L, Vogelaers D, Blot S. Morbidity and mortality of bloodstream infections in patients with severe burn injury. American Journal of Critical Care. 2010;**19**(6):e81–7. DOI: 10.4037/ajcc2010341

[18] Palao R, Monge I, Ruiz M, Barret JP. Chemical burns: Pathophysiology and treatment. Burns. 2010;**36**(3):295–304. DOI: 10.1016/j.burns.2009.07.009

[19] Fish RM, Geddes LA. Conduction of electrical current to and through the human body: A review. Eplasty. 2009;**9**:e44

[20] Arnoldo BD, Purdue GF, Kowalske K, Helm PA, Burris A, Hunt JL. Electrical injuries: A 20-year review. The Journal of Burn Care & Rehabilitation. 2004;**25**(6):479–484. DOI: 10.1097/01.bcr.0000144536.22284.5c

[21] Klein MB, Hayden D, Elson C, Nathens AB, Gamelli RL, Gibran NS, Herndon DN, Arnoldo B, Silver G, Schoenfeld D, Tompkins RG. The association between fluid administration and outcome following major burn: A multicenter study. Annals of Surgery. 2007;**245**(4):622–628. DOI: 10.1097/01.sla.0000252572.50684.49

[22] Branski LK, Gauglitz GG, Herndon DN, Jeschke MG. A review of gene and stem cell therapy in cutaneous wound healing. Burns. 2009;**35**(2):171–180. DOI: 10.1016/j.burns.2008.03.009

[23] Sheridan RL. Burn care for children. Pediatrics in Review. 2018;**39**(6):273–286. DOI: 10.1542/pir.2016-0179

[24] Atiyeh BS, Costagliola M, Hayek SN. Keloid or hypertrophic scar: The controversy: Review of the literature. Annals of Plastic Surgery. 2005;**54**(6):676–680. DOI: 10.1097/01.sap.0000164538.72375.93

[25] Bayat A, McGrouther DA, Ferguson MW. Skin scarring. BMJ. 2003;**326**(7380):88–92. DOI: 10.1136/bmj.326.7380.88

[26] Orgill DP, Blanco C, editors. Biomaterials for Treating Skin Loss. Cambridge: Woodhead Publishing; 2009

[27] Nanchahal J, Dover R, Otto WR. Allogeneic skin substitutes applied to burns patients. Burns. 2002;**28**(3):254–257. DOI: 10.1016/s0305-4179(01)00107-3

[28] Peck MD. Epidemiology of burns throughout the world. Part I: Distribution and risk factors. Burns. 2011;**37**(7):1087–1100. DOI: 10.1016/j.burns.2011.06.005

[29] Sen S, Romanowski K, Miotke S, Palmieri T, Greenhalgh D. Burn prevention in the elderly: Identifying age and gender differences in consumer products associated with burn injuries. Journal of Burn Care & Research. 2021;**42**(1):14–17. DOI: 10.1093/jbcr/iraa175

[30] Yowler CJ, Fratianne RB. Current status of burn resuscitation. Clinics in Plastic Surgery. 2000;**27**(1):1–10

[31] Wood FM, Kolybaba ML, Allen P. The use of cultured epithelial autograft

in the treatment of major burn wounds: Eleven years of clinical experience. Burns. 2006;**32**(5):538–544. DOI: 10.1016/j.burns.2006.02.025

[32] Holmes Iv JH, Molnar JA, Carter JE, Hwang J, Cairns BA, King BT, Smith DJ, Cruse CW, Foster KN, Peck MD, Sood R, Feldman MJ, Jordan MH, Mozingo DW, Greenhalgh DG, Palmieri TL, Griswold JA, Dissanaike S, Hickerson WL. A comparative study of the recell® device and autologous split-thickness meshed skin graft in the treatment of acute burn injuries. Journal of Burn Care & Research. 2018;**39** (5):694–702. DOI: 10.1093/jbcr/iry029

[33] Atiyeh BS. Tissue expansion: A possibly valid reconstructive alternative in electric burns of the mouth. Ann Burns Fire Disasters. 1999;**12**(1):32–35. https://www.medbc.com/annals/review/vol_12/num_1/text/vol12n1p32.htm

[34] Cetin EO, Yesil-Celiktas O, Cavusoglu T, Demirel-Sezer E, Akdemir O, Uyanikgil Y. Incision wound healing activity of pine bark extract containing topical formulations: A study with histopathological and biochemical analyses in albino rats. Die Pharmazie. 2013;**68**(1):75–80

[35] Songur MK, Akdemir O, Lineaweaver WC, Cavusoglu T, Ozsarac M, Aktug H, Songur E, Tiftikcioglu YO. Comparison of skin effects of immediate treatment modalities in experimentally induced hydrofluoric acid skin burns. International Wound Journal. 2015;**12** (6):716–723. DOI: 10.1111/iwj.12214

[36] Hettiaratchy S, Dziewulski P. ABC of burns. Introduction. BMJ. 2004;**328** (7452):1366–1368. DOI: 10.1136/bmj.328.7452.1366

[37] Heimbach DM, Faucher LD. Principles of burn surgery. In: Barret J, Herndon DN, editors. Principles and Practice of Burn Surgery. Boca Raton: CRC Press; 2005. p. 135–162. DOI: 10.1201/b21634

[38] Shupp JW, Nasabzadeh TJ, Rosenthal DS, Jordan MH, Fidler P, Jeng JC. A review of the local pathophysiologic bases of burn wound progression. Journal of Burn Care & Research. 2010;**31**(6):849–873. DOI: 10.1097/BCR.0b013e3181f93571

[39] Singer AJ, Dagum AB. Current management of acute cutaneous wounds. New England Journal of Medicine. 2008;**359**(10):1037–1046. DOI: 10.1056/NEJMra0707253

[40] Sen CK, Gordillo GM, Roy S, Kirsner R, Lambert L, Hunt TK, Gottrup F, Gurtner GC, Longaker MT. Human skin wounds: A major and snowballing threat to public health and the economy. Wound Repair and Regeneration. 2009;**17**(6):763–771. DOI: 10.1111/j.1524-475X.2009.00543.x

[41] Mustoe TA, Cooter RD, Gold MH, Hobbs FD, Ramelet AA, Shakespeare PG, Stella M, Téot L, Wood FM, Ziegler UE. International Advisory Panel on Scar Management. International clinical recommendations on scar management. Plastic and Reconstructive Surgery. 2002;**110** (2):560–571. DOI: 10.1097/00006534-200208000-00031

[42] Gurtner GC, Werner S, Barrandon Y, Longaker MT. Wound repair and regeneration. Nature. 2008;**453**(7193):314–321. DOI: 10.1038/nature07039

[43] Eming SA, Krieg T, Davidson JM. Inflammation in wound repair:

Molecular and cellular mechanisms. Journal of Investigative Dermatology. 2007;**127**(3):514–525. DOI: 10.1038/sj.jid.5700701

[44] Guo S, Dipietro LA. Factors affecting wound healing. Journal of Dental Research. 2010;**89**(3):219–229. DOI: 10.1177/0022034509359125

[45] Sen CK, Roy S. Redox signals in wound healing. Biochimica Et Biophysica Acta (BBA)-General Subjects. 2008;**1780**(11):1348–1361. DOI: 10.1016/j.bbagen.2008.01.006

[46] Peck M, Molnar J, Swart D. A global plan for burn prevention and care. Bulletin of the World Health Organization. 2009;**87**(10):802–803. DOI: 10.2471/blt.08.059733

[47] Williams FN, Herndon DN, Hawkins HK, Lee JO, Cox RA, Kulp GA, Finnerty CC, Chinkes DL, Jeschke MG. The leading causes of death after burn injury in a single pediatric burn center. Critical Care. 2009;**13**(6):R183. DOI: 10.1186/cc8170

[48] Brigham PA, McLoughlin E. Burn incidence and medical care use in the United States: Estimates, trends, and data sources. Journal of Burn Care & Rehabilitation. 1996;**17**(2):95–107. DOI: 10.1097/00004630-199603000-00003

[49] Finnerty CC, Herndon DN, Przkora R, Pereira CT, Oliveira HM, Queiroz DM, Rocha AM, Jeschke MG. Cytokine expression profile over time in severely burned pediatric patients. Shock. 2006;**26**(1):13–19. DOI: 10.1097/01.shk.0000223120.26394.7d

[50] Orgill DP. Excision and skin grafting of thermal burns. New England Journal of Medicine. 2009;**360**(9):893–901. DOI: 10.1056/NEJMct0804451. Erratum in: N Engl J Med. 2011;364(4):389

Section 2

Systemic Responses and Consequences of Burn Injury

Chapter 3

Nutrition in Burn Patients

Ozan Barıs Namdaroglu and Selen Ozturk

Abstract

Burns trigger hypermetabolic and hypercatabolic responses. There is an increase in energy expenditure and nutritional requirements for patients. The developing negative nitrogen balance impairs wound healing and increases the risk of infection and mortality. Nutritional status in burn patients should be assessed early. This assessment should consider clinical factors such as burn surface area, burn depth, age, organ dysfunction, and existing malnutrition. The aim of nutritional therapy is to determine metabolic requirements, preserve lean body mass, and support tissue repair. The gold standard method for determining energy needs is indirect calorimetry. In practical use, mathematical formulas such as Harris–Benedict, Curreri, or Toronto are utilized. However, formulas may not always accurately reflect a patient's actual energy needs. Therefore, energy requirements should not be determined solely on theoretical calculations; the patient's clinical course and metabolic response should be regularly monitored. It should be remembered that both undernutrition and overnutrition can lead to complications. The daily diet for patients should consist of 50–60% carbohydrates, 20–30% lipids, and 1.5–2.0 g/kg protein. Macronutrient distribution should be balanced. Protein supplementation is essential for reducing negative nitrogen balance, preserving muscle mass, and supporting wound healing. We should initiate enteral nutrition as early as possible because of bacterial translocation and gastrointestinal integrity. Early enteral nutrition also contributes to supporting the immune response and reducing infectious complications. In cases where enteral nutrition is insufficient, supplementary parenteral nutrition should be added. In addition, immunonutritional elements such as, glutamine (0.3–0.5 g/kg/day), omega-3 fatty acids, vitamin C, zinc, and selenium are important in improving clinical outcomes because they reduce oxidative stress.

Keywords: burn injury, nutritional support, enteral nutrition, immunonutrition, hypermetabolism

1. Introduction

Severe burn injuries are serious traumas that trigger a prominent metabolic stress response in the organism and lead to numerous systemic changes [1]. In the early period of the burn, metabolic activity increases along with the acute stress response, energy consumption rises, and hemodynamic instability develops. Hypoxia and reperfusion injury occur due to tissue ischemia, and gastrointestinal

IntechOpen

system functions are adversely affected [2, 3]. As a result, significant catabolism develops in severe burns, and patients develop a negative nitrogen balance. Negative nitrogen balance delays wound healing and increases infections and complications [4].

The massive inflammatory reaction and hormonal changes induced by major burns put the organism in a hypermetabolic state. The hypermetabolic state is accompanied by an increase in metabolic rate, rapid metabolism of muscle proteins, suppression of the immune system, and is associated with clinical consequences such as, systemic infections, organ failure, and impaired healing of the wound [1, 5]. Therefore, nutritional support is one of the fundamental approaches for controlling the hypermetabolic response and meeting metabolic requirements. Many factors, such as, total energy requirement, route of feeding, and appropriate distribution of macronutrients, are taken into consideration when planning nutritional therapy in burn patients [6, 7].

The effects of burn injury on nutrition are not limited to the trauma itself. A preexisting state of malnutrition exacerbates the metabolic stress response that develops after a burn. Therefore, the nutritional status of burn patients is evaluated in the early period [8]. In determining nutritional risk, along with the patient's current nutritional status, clinical factors that may affect the course of the disease, such as, the severity of the burn, age, inhalation injury, and organ dysfunction, are also taken into account. The NUTrition Risk in the Critically ill (NUTRIC) score, which is one of the evaluation tools, helps determine the nutritional risk, especially in burn patients treated under intensive care conditions [9].

2. Metabolic and hormonal response in burns

In the postburn period, significant changes occur in energy metabolism and the utilization of nutrients, and there is a marked increase in the nutritional requirements of patients [1, 10]. Although short-term variability is observed in the metabolic rate, a prominent hypermetabolic response usually develops within the first few days. During this process, energy consumption rapidly increases and reaches its peak in most patients within two–three weeks after the injury. It is known that the increase in metabolic rate is generally around 50–80%, and in some patients, it increases up to twofold [1, 10]. Some studies have shown that in severe burn patients, the metabolic rate reaches approximately 1.5–1.7 times normal values [11]. Although the metabolic response decreases over time, it can persist for months or even years in some patients [12].

Postburn metabolism is characterized by catabolic processes. With the increase in inflammatory markers and stress hormones, protein breakdown accelerates, and muscle proteins are used for energy production. Metabolic requirements are met from muscle proteins. This situation causes a negative nitrogen balance, and lean body mass significantly decreases. Due to this catabolic process, wounds heal slowly. Infections and organ dysfunctions occur [13, 14].

Burns also affect carbohydrate and lipid metabolism [1, 10]. Gluconeogenesis and glycolysis increase, lipogenesis is suppressed, and imbalances occur in energy metabolism. Furthermore, the development of insulin resistance impairs the cellular utilization of nutrient substrates, contributing to a further increase in metabolic stress [15].

This situation reveals the importance of nutritional therapy in burn patients. Due to the increased energy requirements and prominent catabolism, appropriate and timely nutritional support is of great importance in terms of meeting metabolic requirements, preserving muscle mass, and supporting wound healing. However, meeting energy requirements solely based on theoretical calculations brings the risk of overfeeding. Overfeeding or rapid feeding practices lead to gastrointestinal intolerance and metabolic complications. Therefore, appropriately evaluating metabolic changes and implementing individualized nutritional strategies in burn patients constitutes an important part of the treatment [7].

3. Assessment of energy requirements

Accurately determining the energy requirement in burn patients is one of the fundamental steps of nutritional therapy. Inadequate energy provision is associated with delayed wound healing, prolonged hospital stay, and an increased risk of complications. Providing excessive energy leads to hyperglycemia, increased carbon dioxide production, and metabolic complications [7, 16].

Indirect calorimetry is the most reliable method for determining energy expenditure in burn patients. It allows for the calculation of the organism's metabolic rate through the measurement of oxygen consumption and carbon dioxide production and is considered the gold standard in determining resting energy expenditure (REE). It accurately calculates the patient's energy requirements and serves as an important guide in planning nutritional therapy [17, 18].

In cases where indirect calorimetry is not feasible, mathematical formulas are used. Numerous formulas have been developed for calculating energy requirements. These formulas generally provide an approximate value [11]. In clinical practice, the Harris–Benedict, Curreri, and Toronto formulas are the most commonly used. Some studies have shown that these formulas may overestimate or underestimate energy requirements. Therefore, it is important to evaluate the calculated values in conjunction with the patient's clinical condition [19, 20].

The patient's age, burn surface area, presence of infection, and surgical history are also important factors in assessing energy requirements. It should be kept in mind that weight changes may occur due to edema developing after fluid replacement. The patient's preinjury body weight should be considered as much as possible when calculating energy requirements [21, 22].

Meeting energy requirements is important for supporting wound healing, reducing the risk of infection, and preserving lean body mass [23]. Excessive energy intake should also be avoided. Specifically, administering calories beyond the target energy requirement can lead to prolonged intubation and metabolic complications due to increased carbon dioxide production. Therefore, energy intake should be monitored regularly. The nutritional plan should be adjusted as needed according to the patient's clinical course [22, 24].

In conclusion, accurately determining energy requirements is a fundamental component of nutritional therapy [24]. Although indirect calorimetry is the most reliable method for assessing energy requirements, formulas are mostly used in clinical practice [17, 18]. Given the limitations of these methods, energy requirements should be assessed in conjunction with clinical monitoring.

4. Macronutrient requirements

In burns, carbohydrates, fats, and proteins are important for energy production, tissue repair, and the maintenance of immune function. Providing patients with these nutrients in appropriate proportions enhances wound healing, preserves muscle mass, and reduces metabolic complications [25, 26].

There is consensus in the literature regarding the protein requirements of burn patients. The daily protein intake should be 1.5–2.0 g/kg or approximately 15–20% of total energy [27, 28]. There are differing opinions on how nonprotein calories should be distributed between carbohydrates and fats.

Most guidelines recommend that approximately 20–30% of total energy should come from fats [29]. Macronutrient ratios may vary depending on the patient's clinical condition, burn surface area, and the nutritional protocol applied [25].

In the past, high-fat diets were used for burn patients. The main rationale for this approach was that fats are high in energy and lead to lower carbon dioxide production compared to carbohydrates [30]. However, subsequent studies have shown that high lipid intake can lead to adverse metabolic outcomes, such as, hyperlipidemia, hepatic fat accumulation, and suppression of immune functions [15]. Today, lipid intake in burn patients is planned more balanced, and macronutrient distribution is adjusted according to the metabolic state of the patient [31].

In recent years, the importance of carbohydrates in burn nutrition has been emphasized more, particularly due to their nitrogen-sparing effects. Therefore, nutritional formulations containing relatively low fat and higher carbohydrates are preferred in some burn centers [25]. However, it is not recommended to reduce lipid intake excessively. Nutritional regimens containing very low fat can lead to essential fatty acid deficiency, just as excessive carbohydrate intake increases the risk of hyperglycemia [15, 32, 33]. Therefore, macronutrient distribution must be planned in a balanced manner in accordance with the patient's clinical condition and metabolic requirements.

4.1 Protein metabolism and requirement

Following the systemic inflammatory response and the effect of stress hormones that develop after a burn injury, marked protein catabolism occurs in the organism. Especially skeletal muscle proteins are rapidly degraded, and a large amount of free amino acids is released into the circulation. These amino acids are used in the synthesis of collagen, which plays a role in the synthesis of acute-phase proteins, the maintenance of the immune response, and wound healing [34]. Amino acids contribute to meeting the organism's energy requirements by providing substrates for gluconeogenesis [35].

During periods of hypermetabolic response, protein catabolism is prominent and often exceeds the rate of protein synthesis. In severely burned patients, daily protein breakdown reaches approximately 150–250 g. This is associated with a significant decrease in muscle mass and a negative nitrogen balance. A negative nitrogen balance impairs wound healing, suppresses immune function, and increases the risk of infection [34, 35].

Providing adequate protein support in burn patients is one of the fundamental components of nutritional therapy. Increased catabolism, protein synthesis necessary for wound healing, and the maintenance of immune functions are the main reasons for the increased protein requirement. Current guidelines recommend planning protein intake at a level of 1.5–2.0 g/kg daily, and this approach contributes to reducing protein catabolism and preserving lean body mass [28].

4.2 Carbohydrate metabolism

Burns cause changes in the amount of carbohydrates the body uses. Initially, the body rapidly consumes the carbohydrates it has stored. Then, it begins to produce glucose through gluconeogenesis. Insulin resistance develops in patients, which disrupts the transport and metabolism of glucose in the body [36].

Mitochondrial dysfunction and changes in oxidative phosphorylation affect glucose metabolism. This reduces the efficient use of glucose in energy production and causes an increase in energy consumption [36]. To meet the increased energy requirement, the organism begins to rely more on the glycolysis pathway. Excessive glycolysis leads to lactic acid accumulation. Patients should be carefully monitored in this regard [37].

Sufficient carbohydrate intake reduces protein catabolism. Sufficient carbohydrate intake is effective in maintaining nitrogen balance. Carbohydrates are the main energy source in burn patients. Sufficient carbohydrate intake reduces protein breakdown [38].

4.3 Lipid metabolism

Burns also cause changes in lipid metabolism. Oxidation of free fatty acids from adipose tissue increases during the postburn period. These oxidized fatty acids are utilized to meet the increased energy requirements. Lipids also contribute to the synthesis of certain hormones and inflammatory mediators [38].

Burns lead to a decrease in apolipoprotein and carnitine synthesis. Mitochondrial oxidation of fatty acids is impaired, and lipid metabolism disorders occur [39]. Some of the unusable fatty acids accumulate in the liver in the form of triglycerides, leading to the development of hepatomegaly and hepatosteatosis [40].

Consumption of lipids in patients with burns must be approached with utmost caution and care. Fats are a significant source of energy, but if the intake of lipids is excessive, it may lead to metabolic complications. It is, therefore, advisable to modify lipid intake based on the patient's metabolic condition and clinical tolerance [38].

5. Micronutrients and immunonutrition

The hypermetabolic and inflammatory response that develops after major burn injuries not only increases energy and macronutrient requirements but also affects the need for vitamins, trace elements, and immunomodulatory nutrients. Extensive burn surface area, losses through wound exudate, increased oxidative stress, and increased requirements in tissue repair lead to the development of micronutrient deficiencies. These deficiencies are associated with delays in wound healing, increased infection risk, and impairments in immune functions. Evaluating micronutrients and immunonutrients in burn patients and supplementing them in appropriate situations is one of the important components of nutritional therapy [41].

5.1 Immunonutrients (glutamine, arginine, and omega-3 fatty acids)

Although glutamine is a nonessential amino acid under physiological conditions, it becomes "conditionally essential" in critical illness situations such as, severe trauma, major surgery, and extensive burns. The hypermetabolic and hypercatabolic response developing after a burn increases glutamine consumption, and a significant decrease in plasma glutamine levels is observed. In addition, losses through wound exudate also contribute to the depletion of glutamine stores [42].

Glutamine is an important energy source for the intestinal mucosa and plays a role in preserving the integrity of the intestinal barrier. Glutamine supplementation is beneficial in terms of preserving the intestinal mucosa, reducing bacterial translocation, and modulating the inflammatory response. Some clinical studies have reported that glutamine supplementation reduces infection rates and limits protein catabolism. It is also stated in larger-scale studies that this benefit could not be consistently demonstrated in all patients. Current guidelines recommend glutamine supplementation at a dose of approximately 0.3–0.5 g/kg/day after starting enteral nutrition in patients with extensive burns [42].

Arginine and omega-3 fatty acids are other immunomodulatory nutrients investigated in burn patients. Arginine is an amino acid that plays a role in the regulation of the immune response and wound healing processes. Evidence regarding its routine use in critically ill patients and in situations with a risk of sepsis is limited, and its application is evaluated according to patient characteristics [3].

Long-chain omega-3 fatty acids are known for their antiinflammatory and immunomodulatory effects. It has been reported that fish oil-based enteral nutritional formulations, containing especially eicosapentaenoic acid (EPA) and docosahexaenoic acid (DHA), reduce the postburn inflammatory response and regulate immune functions. Some studies have shown that enteral nutrition containing omega-3 fatty acids reduces infection rates and improves clinical outcomes. The available data are heterogeneous, and the use of these nutrients is evaluated in accordance with the patient's clinical condition and nutritional requirements [43, 44].

5.2 Vitamins

Preserving the normal metabolism of numerous vitamins and trace elements is important after a burn because these micronutrients play a critical role in the maintenance of the immune response and wound healing processes. Major burn injuries lead to pronounced oxidative stress, developing along with a strong inflammatory response, and this process increases the consumption of micronutrients involved in antioxidant defense systems [41].

Vitamin C is of fundamental importance in terms of collagen synthesis, wound healing, and antioxidant defense mechanisms. It has been shown that vitamin C consumption increases in burn patients, and its supplementation contributes to wound healing by supporting collagen formation. It also contributes to reducing the risk of infection by supporting immune functions [45].

Vitamin A stimulates epithelial cell growth, thereby supporting re-epithelialization, and plays a role in regulating the immune response. Its deficiency leads to impaired collagen synthesis and delayed wound healing. However, due to its stores in the liver, pronounced systemic deficiency is not seen in every patient [46].

Vitamin D plays an important role in regulating bone metabolism, and low levels are frequently reported in burn patients. Nevertheless, the clinical effects of vitamin D deficiency after severe burns and the optimal supplementation doses are not yet completely clear [47].

Although vitamin E has also demonstrated wound-healing supportive effects in some studies due to its antioxidant properties, vitamin supplementation should be planned in accordance with the patient's clinical condition and laboratory findings rather than being routinely applied to every patient [46].

5.3 Trace elements

Trace element metabolism is also significantly affected in burn patients. Extensive burn surface area and losses through wound exudate lead to a decrease in the levels of elements such as, zinc, copper, and selenium. In addition, the distribution of trace elements within the body may change during the acute phase response [48].

Zinc is an important trace element for wound healing, DNA synthesis, protein synthesis, and immune cell functions. A significant amount of zinc loss occurs from burn wounds via exudate. Zinc deficiency is associated with impaired immune functions and delayed wound healing. Therefore, adequate zinc supplementation supports wound healing [49].

Selenium has strong antioxidant properties and is found in the structure of many antioxidant enzymes, especially glutathione peroxidase. A decrease in serum selenium levels can be seen in burn patients, and this condition contributes to an increase in oxidative stress. There are data indicating that appropriate selenium supplementation can reduce infectious complications [50].

Copper is an important trace element required for collagen synthesis, immune functions, and hematopoiesis. In burn patients, copper metabolism is affected due to mineral losses occurring with wound exudate. A decrease in serum copper levels can be seen in patients with extensive burns, and this situation may be associated with delayed wound healing, anemia, and immune dysfunction. Monitoring copper levels in patients with extensive burns is important [51].

Iron metabolism undergoes complex changes in burn patients. A temporary increase in serum iron levels is observed due to hemolysis in the early period of the burn injury. However, in the later period, iron utilization disorders and anemia develop under the influence of the inflammatory response and regulatory mechanisms in iron metabolism. Iron supplementation should not be routinely administered to every burn patient; it should be evaluated individually based on the clinical condition and laboratory findings [51].

5.4 Other minerals

Significant changes are also seen in calcium, magnesium, and phosphorus metabolism in burn patients. In particular, a decrease in phosphorus levels may develop in the early postburn period, and this condition should be closely monitored at the beginning of nutritional therapy. Hypomagnesemia is associated with neuromuscular irritability and cardiac rhythm disturbances. Changes in calcium metabolism can lead to bone resorption and disruption of mineral balance, especially in pediatric patients. Since changes in electrolyte and mineral levels are associated with fluid resuscitation, the inflammatory response, and metabolic stress, regular laboratory monitoring is important [51].

5.5 Clinical approach

Micronutrients and immunonutrients play an important role in wound healing, the preservation of immune functions, and the reduction of oxidative stress in burn patients. It should be kept in mind that not all supplements provide the same level of benefit to every patient. The most appropriate approach is the application of a personalized nutritional strategy by evaluating the clinical condition, burn surface area, metabolic requirements, and laboratory findings together. Regular clinical and biochemical monitoring with a multidisciplinary approach is of fundamental importance in determining the appropriate micronutrient support.

Table 1 shows nutritional goals and recommended parameters in burn patients.

6. Enteral and parenteral nutrition

The current approach is to start enteral nutrition as soon as possible in order to benefit from the physiological functions of the gastrointestinal tract and to support it with parenteral nutrition when necessary [52].

In order to plan nutritional therapy for burn patients, it is important to determine the nutritional risk in the early period. One of the screening tools commonly used in clinical practice is the Nutritional Risk Screening-2002 (NRS-2002). This method aims to determine whether patients need nutritional support by evaluating parameters such as, body mass index, weight loss, decrease in food intake, and disease severity. However, it is known that disease-specific factors, such as, total burn surface area and burn depth, also significantly affect nutritional status in burn patients. Some studies have proposed modified evaluation models that also include these parameters. These approaches contribute to a more comprehensive evaluation of nutritional risk in burn patients and the determination of an appropriate nutritional strategy [53].

6.1 Early enteral nutrition

Early enteral nutrition is considered a fundamental approach to nutritional therapy. Guidelines recommend initiating enteral nutrition as soon as possible in hemodynamically stable patients, ideally within the first 24 hours after a burn [54].

Parameter	Method/recommendation	Note
Energy (gold standard)	Indirect calorimetry	It is the most reliable method for determining resting energy expenditure (REE).
Estimated formulas	Harris–Benedict, Curreri, or Toronto Formulas	Provides an approximate value in situations where calorimetry cannot be performed
Protein requirement	1.5–2.0 g/kg/day	Critical for preventing negative nitrogen balance and preserving muscle mass
Carbohydrate	Approximately 50–60% of total energy	Provides protein-sparing and is the main energy source
Lipid	20–30% of total energy	Excessive lipid intake (risk of hepatic steatosis) should be avoided
Glutamine support	0.3–0.5 g/kg/day	Recommended for extensive burns.

Table 1.
Nutritional goals and recommended parameters in burn patients.

Hypoperfusion and systemic inflammatory response resulting from burns cause ischemic changes in the mucosal lining of the gastrointestinal tract. This impairs the integrity and barrier function of the mucosa. Bacterial translocation occurs. Early initiation of enteral nutrition trophically stimulates the intestinal mucosa and helps prevent complications. Maintaining intestinal barrier function is crucial for supporting the immune system and reducing the risk of infection [55].

Numerous articles have shown that early enteral nutrition reduces the incidence of sepsis and gastrointestinal bleeding and shortens hospital stays. Furthermore, it is believed that contact between food and the intestinal mucosa contributes to the preservation of mucosal integrity and the maintenance of the gut microbiota. These are considered fundamental physiological processes that explain the positive effects of early enteral nutrition on clinical outcomes [56].

6.2 Enteral feeding intolerance

Early enteral nutrition is recommended after burns, but the gastrointestinal system is frequently affected in severe burns. In the early stages, mucosal ischemia, edema, and motility disorders can occur in the gastrointestinal system, reducing enteral nutrition tolerance. Studies show that enteral nutrition intolerance ranges from approximately 30–70% in patients with severe burns. Intolerance generally develops within two weeks of injury. Risk factors for feeding intolerance include a large burned surface area, low blood pressure, high blood sugar levels, and gastrointestinal dysfunction [57].

In cases of enteral feeding intolerance, symptoms such as, vomiting, abdominal distension, increased gastric emptying volume, and decreased bowel sounds may occur. Methods considered include reducing the feeding rate, using prokinetic drugs, or switching to postpyloric feeding. Early diagnosis and proper management of enteral feeding intolerance are very important because they are associated with a poor prognosis [58].

Duodenal or jejunal feeding should be considered in cases of enteral feeding intolerance. Jejunal feeding reduces the risk of aspiration and gastroesophageal reflux. It is especially preferred in patients with a high risk of aspiration or in the presence of marked gastroparesis. It has been reported that jejunal feeding increases intestinal microcirculation and contributes to the preservation of gastrointestinal functions. While administering jejunal feeding, the patient's clinical condition should be carefully monitored and feeding tolerance should be evaluated regularly [59].

6.3 Parenteral nutrition

Although enteral nutrition is the preferred feeding method in burn patients, it is not sufficient on its own in some clinical situations. Parenteral nutrition is used as an important supportive method, especially in situations where gastrointestinal functions are severely impaired or target energy requirements cannot be met with enteral nutrition [3, 60].

Current approaches emphasize that enteral and parenteral nutrition should be evaluated not as alternative methods to each other but as complementary strategies. In cases where enteral nutrition is not possible, or adequate energy and protein intake cannot be achieved with enteral nutrition, supplemental parenteral nutrition is applied. This approach helps meet the patient's metabolic requirements while reducing the risk of prolonged fasting and malnutrition [3, 60].

Long-term parenteral nutrition is associated with some adverse effects, such as, gastrointestinal mucosal atrophy, catheter-related infections, metabolic complications, and hepatic dysfunction. Therefore, parenteral nutrition should be applied with careful patient selection, and transition to enteral nutrition should be targeted as soon as possible [57, 61].

In conclusion, nutritional therapy in burn patients is a dynamic process and should be planned considering the patient's clinical condition, gastrointestinal functions, and metabolic requirements. Initiating enteral nutrition, if possible, within the first 24 hours after injury should be considered the fundamental approach. Supporting it with supplemental parenteral nutrition, when necessary, is important for optimal nutrition management [3, 7, 57].

7. Conclusion

Burn injury creates a marked hypermetabolic and hypercatabolic response in the organism, leading to significant increases in energy and nutrient requirements. Appropriate nutritional support is one of the fundamental components of burn treatment. Nutrition management in burn patients includes correctly determining the energy requirements, providing a balanced supply of macro and micronutrients, and selecting the appropriate route of feeding.

The current approach is to start enteral nutrition as early as possible and to support it with supplemental parenteral nutrition in necessary situations. Individualized nutritional strategies, planned by considering the patient's clinical condition, metabolic requirements, and feeding tolerance, significantly contribute to reducing complications and improving clinical outcomes in burn patients.

Furthermore, it should not be ignored that the healing process in burn injuries does not end with the hospitalization period. Increased metabolic needs, which can continue for months during the postdischarge rehabilitation phase, scar maturation, and the regaining of lost lean body mass necessitate long-term and structured outpatient nutritional monitoring.

Acknowledgments

The authors acknowledge the use of ChatGPT for language editing in the chapter.

Author details

Ozan Barıs Namdaroglu* and Selen Ozturk
Tepecik Training and Research Hospital, General Surgery Clinic, Izmir, Türkiye

*Address all correspondence to: ozannamdaroglu@yahoo.com

References

[1] Clark A, Imran J, Madni T, Wolf SE. Nutrition and metabolism in burn patients. Burns & Trauma. 2017;**5**:11. DOI: 10.1186/s41038-017-0076-x

[2] Rousseau AF, Pantet O, Heyland DK. Nutrition after severe burn injury. Current Opinion in Clinical Nutrition and Metabolic Care. 2023;**26**(2):99–104. DOI: 10.1097/MCO.0000000000000904

[3] Singer P, Blaser AR, Berger MM, et al. ESPEN guideline on clinical nutrition in the intensive care unit. Clinical Nutrition (Edinburgh, Scotland). 2019;**38**(1):48–79. DOI: 10.1016/j.clnu.2018.08.037

[4] Prelack K, Dylewski M, Sheridan RL. Practical guidelines for nutritional management of burn injury and recovery. Burns. 2007;**33**(1):14–24. DOI: 10.1016/j.burns.2006.06.014

[5] Moreira E, Burghi G, Manzanares W. Update on metabolism and nutrition therapy in critically ill burn patients. Medicina Intensiva. 2018;**42**(5):306–316. DOI: 10.1016/j.medin.2017.07.007

[6] Oryan A, Alemzadeh E, Moshiri A. Burn wound healing: Present concepts, treatment strategies and future directions. Journal of Wound Care. 2017;**26**(1):5–19. DOI: 10.12968/jowc.2017.26.1.5

[7] Rousseau AF, Losser MR, Ichai C, Berger MM. ESPEN endorsed recommendations: Nutritional therapy in major burns. Clinical Nutrition. 2013;**32**(4):497–502. DOI: 10.1016/j.clnu.2013.02.012

[8] Caldis-Coutris N, Gawaziuk JP, Magnusson S, et al. Malnutrition in burns: A prospective, single-center study. Journal of Burn Care & Research. 2022;**43**(3):592–595. DOI: 10.1093/jbcr/irab186

[9] Bang YK, Park MK, Ju YS, Cho KY. Clinical significance of nutritional risk screening tool for hospitalised children with acute burn injuries: A cross-sectional study. Journal of Human Nutrition and Dietetics. 2018;**31**(3):370–378. DOI: 10.1111/jhn.12518

[10] Peng X. New perspective on clinical nutrition in burn injuries. Zhonghua Shao Shang Za Zhi = Zhonghua Shaoshang Zazhi = Chinese Journal of Burns. 2019;**35**(5):321–325. DOI: 10.3760/cma.j.issn.1009-2587.2019.05.001

[11] Dickerson RN, Gervasio JM, Riley ML, et al. Accuracy of predictive methods to estimate resting energy expenditure of thermally-injured patients. Journal of Parenteral and Enteral Nutrition. 2002;**26**(1):17–29. DOI: 10.1177/014860710202600117

[12] Porter C, Herndon DN, Børsheim E, et al. Long-term skeletal muscle mitochondrial dysfunction is associated with hypermetabolism in severely burned children. Journal of Burn Care & Research. 2016;**37**(1):53–63. DOI: 10.1097/BCR.0000000000000308

[13] Porter C, Herndon DN, Bhattarai N, et al. Severe burn injury induces thermogenically functional mitochondria in murine white adipose tissue. Shock. 2015;**44**(3):258–264. DOI: 10.1097/SHK.0000000000000410

[14] Hart DW, Wolf SE, Mlcak R, et al. Persistence of muscle catabolism after severe burn. Surgery. 2000;**128**(2):312–319. DOI: 10.1067/msy.2000.108059

[15] Demling RH, Seigne P. Metabolic management of patients with severe burns. World Journal of Surgery. 2000;**24**(6):673–680. DOI: 10.1007/s002689910109

[16] Chourdakis M, Bouras E, Shields BA, Stoppe C, Rousseau AF, Heyland DK. Nutritional therapy among burn injured patients in the critical care setting: An international multicenter observational study on "best achievable" practices. Clinical Nutrition. 2020;**39**(12):3813–3820. DOI: 10.1016/j.clnu.2020.04.023

[17] Leung J, Ridley EJ, Cleland H, et al. Predictive energy equations are inaccurate for determining energy expenditure in adult burn injury: A retrospective observational study. ANZ Journal of Surgery. 2019;**89**(5):578–583. DOI: 10.1111/ans.15119

[18] Delsoglio M, Achamrah N, Berger MM, et al. Indirect calorimetry in clinical practice. Journal of Clinical Medicine. 2019;**8**(9):1387. DOI: 10.3390/jcm8091387

[19] Jeon J, Kym D, Cho YS, et al. Reliability of resting energy expenditure in major burns: Comparison between measured and predictive equations. Clinical Nutrition. 2019;**38**(6):2763–2769. DOI: 10.1016/j.clnu.2018.12.003

[20] Guo F, Zhou H, Wu J, et al. Prospective study on energy expenditure in patients with severe burns. Journal of Parenteral and Enteral Nutrition. 2021;**45**(1):146–151. DOI: 10.1002/jpen.1819

[21] Chan LC, Lee MS, Ou YN, et al. Energy requirements for ICU burn patients in whom the total body surface area affected exceeds 50 percent: A practical equation. Asia Pacific Journal of Clinical Nutrition. 2018;**27**(6):1182–1189. DOI: 10.6133/apjcn.201811_27(6).0003

[22] Gottschlich MM, editor. A.S.P.E.N. Nutrition Support Core Curriculum: A Case-Based Approach-the Adult Patient. Silver Spring, MD: American Society for Parenteral and Enteral Nutrition; 2007. p. 405–423

[23] Saffle JR, Larson CM, Sullivan J. A randomized trial of indirect calorimetry-based feedings in thermal injury. The Journal of Trauma: Injury, Infection, and Critical Care. 1990;**30**(6):776–783. DOI: 10.1097/00005373-199007000-00003

[24] Shields BA, Doty KA, Chung KK, Wade CE, Aden JK, Wolf SE. Determination of resting energy expenditure after severe burn. Journal of Burn Care & Research. 2013;**34**(1):e22–e28. DOI: 10.1097/BCR.0b013e318254d2d5

[25] Shields BA, VanFosson CA, Pruskowski KA, Gurney JM, Rizzo JA, Cancio LC. High-Carbohydrate vs High-Fat Nutrition for Burn Patients. Nutrition in Clinical Practice. 2019;**34**(5):688–694. DOI: 10.1002/ncp.10396

[26] Hew JJ, Parungao RJ, Tsai KH, et al. The geometric framework reveals that moderate protein, high carbohydrate intake is optimal for severe burn injury in mice. British Journal of Nutrition. 2020;**123**(9):1056–1067. DOI: 10.1017/S0007114520000276

[27] Wise AK, Hromatka KA, Miller KR. Energy expenditure and protein

requirements following burn injury. Nutrition in Clinical Practice. 2019;**34**(5):673–680. DOI: 10.1002/ncp.10390

[28] McClave SA, Taylor BE, Martindale RG, et al. Guidelines for the provision and assessment of nutrition support therapy in the adult critically ill patient: Society of Critical Care Medicine (SCCM) and American Society for Parenteral and Enteral Nutrition (A.S.P.E.N.). Journal of Parenteral and Enteral Nutrition. 2016;**40**(2):159–211. DOI: 10.1177/0148607115621863

[29] Berger MM. Basics in clinical nutrition: Nutritional support in burn patients. E-SPEN, the European e-Journal of Clinical Nutrition and Metabolism. 2009;**4**(6):e308–e312. DOI: 10.1016/j.eclnm.2009.06.005

[30] Lee JO, Gauglitz GG, Herndon DN, et al. Association between dietary fat content and outcomes in pediatric burn patients. Journal of Surgical Research. 2011;**166**(2):e83–e90. DOI: 10.1016/j.jss.2010.10.006

[31] Masters B, Aarabi S, Sidhwa F, Wood F. High-carbohydrate, high-protein, low-fat versus low-carbohydrate, high-protein, high-fat enteral feeds for burns. The Cochrane Database of Systematic Reviews. 2012;**1**:CD006122. DOI: 10.1002/14651858.CD006122.pub3

[32] Newsholme EA, Calder PC, Yaqoob P. The regulatory, informational, and immunomodulatory roles of fat fuels. The American Journal of Clinical Nutrition. 1993;**57**(5 Suppl): 738S–751S. DOI: 10.1093/ajcn/57.5.738S

[33] DeBiasse MA, Wilmore DW.What is optimal nutritional support? New Horizons (Baltimore, Md.). 1994;**2**(2):122–130

[34] Peng X. Further understanding of the hypermetabolism mechanism in burn injury and the strategy of regulation and control. Chinese Journal of Burns. 2013;**29**(2):139–143. DOI: 10.3760/cma.j.issn.1009-2587.2013.02.012

[35] Knuth CM, Auger C, Jeschke MG. Burn-induced hypermetabolism and skeletal muscle dysfunction. American Journal of Physiology-Cell Physiology. 2021;**321**(1):C58–C71. DOI: 10.1152/ajpcell.00106.2021

[36] Xu HZ, Yu YM, Ma H, et al. Glucose metabolism during the early "flow phase" after burn injury. Journal of Surgical Research. 2013;**179**(1):e83–e90. DOI: 10.1016/j.jss.2012.02.037

[37] Badoiu SC, Miricescu D, Stanescu-Spinu II, et al. Glucose metabolism in burns-What happens? International Journal of Molecular Sciences. 2021;**22**(10):5159. DOI: 10.3390/ijms22105159

[38] Clayton RP, Herndon DN, Abate N, Porter C. Impact of burn trauma on lipid and glucose metabolism: Implications for insulin sensitivity. Journal of Burn Care & Research. 2018;**39**(5):713–723. DOI: 10.1093/jbcr/irx047

[39] Gauglitz GG, Finnerty CC, Herndon DN, Williams FN, Jeschke MG. Chapter 30-Modulation of the hypermetabolic response after burn injury. In: Herndon DN, editor. Total Burn Care. 4th ed. Philadelphia (PA): W.B. Saunders; 2012. p. 355–360. DOI: 10.1016/B978-1-4377-2786-9.00030-8

[40] Jeschke MG, Chinkes DL, Finnerty CC, et al. Pathophysiologic response to severe burn injury. Annals

of Surgery. 2008;**248**(3):387–401. DOI: 10.1097/SLA.0b013e3181856241

[41] Berger MM. Antioxidant micronutrients in major trauma and burns: Evidence and practice. Nutrition in Clinical Practice. 2006;**21**(5): 438–449. DOI: 10.1177/0115426506021005438

[42] Singer P, Blaser AR, Berger MM, et al. ESPEN practical and partially revised guideline: Clinical nutrition in the intensive care unit. Clinical Nutrition. 2023;**42**(9):1671–1689. DOI: 10.1016/j.clnu.2023.07.011

[43] Koekkoek WAK, Panteleon V, van Zanten ARH. Current evidence on omega-3 fatty acids in enteral nutrition in the critically ill: A systematic review and meta-analysis. Nutrition. 2019;**59**:56–68. DOI: 10.1016/j.nut.2018.07.013

[44] Calder PC, Yaqoob P. Omega-3 polyunsaturated fatty acids and human health outcomes. Biofactors. 2009;**35** (3):266–272. DOI: 10.1002/biof.42

[45] Carr AC, Maggini S. Vitamin C and immune function. Nutrients. 2017;**9** (11):1211. DOI: 10.3390/nu9111211

[46] Rock CL, Dechert RE, Khilnani R, Parker RS, Rodriguez JL. Carotenoids and antioxidant vitamins in patients after burn injury. The Journal of Burn Care & Rehabilitation. 1997;**18**(3):269–278. DOI: 10.1097/00004630-199705000-00018

[47] Klein GL, Herndon DN, Chen TC, Kulp G, Holick MF. Standard multivitamin supplementation does not improve burn-induced vitamin D deficiency. Journal of Bone and Mineral Metabolism. 2009;**27**:502–506. DOI: 10.1007/s00774-009-0065-7

[48] Berger MM, Reintam-Blaser A, Calder PC, et al. Monitoring nutrition in the ICU. Clinical Nutrition. 2019;**38** (2):584–593. DOI: 10.1016/j.clnu.2018.07.009

[49] Maares M, Haase H. Zinc and immunity: An essential interrelation. Archives of Biochemistry and Biophysics. 2016;**611**:58–65. DOI: 10.1016/j.abb.2016.03.022

[50] Kurmis R, Greenwood J, Aromataris E. Trace element supplementation following severe burn injury: A systematic review and meta-analysis. Journal of Burn Care & Research. 2016;**37**(3):143–159. DOI: 10.1097/BCR.0000000000000259

[51] Gutowska I, Zwierzchowski W, Piorun K, et al. The extent of burn injury significantly affects serum micro- and macroelement concentrations in patients on the first day of hospitalisation. Nutrients. 2022;**14** (20):4248. DOI: 10.3390/nu14204248

[52] Gungabissoon U, Hacquoil K, Bains C, et al. Prevalence, risk factors, clinical consequences, and treatment of enteral feed intolerance during critical illness. Journal of Parenteral and Enteral Nutrition. 2015;**39**(4):441–448. DOI: 10.1177/0148607114526450

[53] Alfonso-Ortiz L, Jiang X, Turgeon AF, et al. Validation of the modified NUTrition Risk Score (mNUTRIC) in mechanically ventilated, severe burn patients: A prospective multinational cohort study. Burns. 2021;**47**(8):1739–1747. DOI: 10.1016/j.burns.2021.05.010

[54] Gottschlich MM, Jenkins ME, Mayes T, Khoury J, Kagan RJ, Warden GD. The 2002 Clinical Research Award. An evaluation of the safety of

early vs delayed enteral support and effects on clinical, nutritional, and endocrine outcomes after severe burns. The Journal of Burn Care & Rehabilitation. 2002;**23**(6):401–415. DOI: 10.1097/01.BCR.0000036588.09166.F1

[55] McClave SA, Heyland DK. The physiologic response and associated clinical benefits from provision of early enteral nutrition. Nutrition in Clinical Practice. 2009;**24**(3):305–315. DOI: 10.1177/0884533609335176

[56] Pu H, Doig GS, Heighes PT, et al. Early enteral nutrition reduces mortality and improves other key outcomes in patients with major burn injury: A meta-analysis of randomized controlled trials. Critical Care Medicine. 2018;**46**(12):2036–2042. DOI: 10.1097/CCM.0000000000003445

[57] Guo F, Zhou H, Wu J, et al. A prospective observation on nutrition support in adult patients with severe burns. British Journal of Nutrition. 2019;**121**(9):974–981. DOI: 10.1017/S0007114519000217

[58] Pan Y, Xu S, Fan Y, et al. Analysis of risk factors of early enteral nutrition intolerance in extremely severe burn patients. Zhonghua Shao Shang Yu Chuang Mian Xiu Fu Za Zhi. 2021;**37**(9). DOI: 10.3760/cma.j.cn501120-20210511-00180

[59] Kurmis R, Nicholls C, Singer Y, et al. An investigation of the provision of early enteral nutrition in major burn patients in Australia and New Zealand. Nutrition & Dietetics. 2022;**79**(5):582–589. DOI: 10.1111/1747-0080.12746

[60] Russell MK, Wischmeyer PE. Supplemental parenteral nutrition: Review of the literature and current nutrition guidelines. Nutrition in Clinical Practice. 2018;**33**(3):359–369. DOI: 10.1002/ncp.10096

[61] Gavin NC, Larsen E, Runnegar N, et al. Association between intravenous lipid emulsion containing parenteral nutrition and bloodstream infections in patients with single-lumen central venous access: A secondary analysis of a randomized trial. Journal of Parenteral and Enteral Nutrition. 2023;**47**(6):783–795. DOI: 10.1002/jpen.2530

Chapter 4

Autophagy/Mitophagy Dysregulation and Neuroimmune Crosstalk in Burn-Induced Skeletal Muscle Dysfunction: Mechanistic Insights and Therapeutic Prospects

Shingo E. Yasuhara, Zerong You, Diroji Antony and Takahiko Tamura

Abstract

Severe thermal injury may induce a prolonged state of metabolic and inflammatory stress, resulting in skeletal muscle dysregulation. Mitochondrial dysfunction and autophagy/mitophagy dysregulations are important features of burn-induced skeletal muscle pathology, with literature presenting altered regulation in both directions. This seeming contradiction may result from approaches that highlight snapshot assessments of the basal state, which do not reflect the dynamic, stress-responsive adaptive capacity. This chapter argues that burn-related skeletal muscle dysfunction is best evidenced as a defect in adaptive mitochondrial quality control rather than an up- or downregulation of autophagic flux. Skeletal muscles in critical illnesses appear to maintain basal autophagy/mitophagy at normal levels but fail to mount an adequate, stress-coupled response to metabolic and inflammatory insult. Framing the problem in this way helps reconcile discordant findings across the literature and situates intrinsic mitochondrial vulnerability within the broader context of neuroimmune-metabolic stress signaling. We suggest that the underlying pathophysiology is driven less by a fixed defect in any one pathway than by a bidirectional amplification between muscle-intrinsic maladaptation and the systemic stress load, a distinction that has meaningful consequences for how we interpret experimental data. Therapeutic approaches may need to prioritize restoring stress-responsive mitochondrial resilience over non-selective activation of autophagy pathways. Distinguishing basal activity and adaptive responsiveness has important implications for translational research and drug discovery. An alternative systems-level perspective combining metabolic, mitochondrial, and neuroimmune regulation may offer a more unifying approach for augmenting long-term functional recovery following severe burn injury.

IntechOpen

Keywords: autophagy, mitophagy, burn injury, skeletal muscle, mitochondrial dysfunction, neuroimmune crosstalk, metabolic stress, adaptive responsiveness

1. Introduction

Severe thermal injury is now considered not only a local tissue damage but also a systemic disease with profound metabolic and inflammatory responses [1, 2]. Among the organs implicated, skeletal muscle is a key determinant of long-term functional outcomes following injury. Despite the evolution of acute care to improve survival, many key challenges remain: persistent muscle weakness, delayed rehabilitation, and chronic morbidity in burn survivors [3, 4]. These clinical observations suggest that burn-induced muscle dysfunction is a form of persistent dysregulation indicative of an adaptive homeostasis disturbance beyond acute transient metabolic derangements [1, 5–9].

The burn environment extracts a chronic hypermetabolic response: increased energy expenditure, insulin resistance, inflammatory activation, and oxidative stress [7, 10]. Skeletal muscle is in a constant state of catabolic pressure in this scenario. Under homeostatic conditions, muscle preserves structural and metabolic integrity via fully coordinated protein turnover and mitochondrial remodeling. The ability of skeletal muscle to maintain adaptive capacity under repeated stress is not merely a reflection of resilience; it is itself a central determinant of whether pathological amplification occurs [11].

At the heart of this adaptive network are mitochondria. They also integrate beyond ATP production to redox signaling, metabolic flux, inflammatory responses, and apoptotic pathways [12]. Their integrity relies on a balance between biogenesis, fission-fusion dynamics, and selective degradation via mitophagy. Mitochondria resemble powerful energy reactors: essential for cellular survival yet potentially hazardous when damaged. Eukaryotic cells have evolved sophisticated containment systems to manage this risk, with autophagy and mitophagy serving as core quality control mechanisms conserved from yeast to humans. It is now well established that this quality control machinery is disrupted in the muscle pathology of many human diseases [13–15], including critical illnesses, but how it is disrupted remains contested [16–19]. Reports of both increased and decreased autophagy and mitophagy activity have accumulated without resolution.

We argue that this inconsistency is partly methodological. Static measurements taken under resting conditions are poorly suited to evaluating mechanisms that exist precisely to respond to stress. In a disease defined by sustained metabolic and inflammatory challenges, what matters is not the baseline activity of a pathway but whether that pathway can respond appropriately when called upon.

This chapter proposes a reframing: autophagy and mitophagy dysregulation in burn-injured skeletal muscle is best understood as a failure of adaptive mitochondrial quality control rather than as a fixed increase or decrease in pathway activity. Impaired stress-responsive mitophagy, we argue, offers a potential explanation for the conflicting findings in the literature. This perspective connects systemic metabolic stress, intrinsic mitochondrial vulnerability, and neuroimmune-metabolic signaling into a single model of muscle vulnerability [20]. The therapeutic implications follow accordingly: the goal is to restore adaptive capacity, not to normalize isolated pathway markers.

2. Metabolomic profiles of skeletal muscle under thermal injury-mediated metabolic stress

2.1 Systemic metabolic stress following severe burns

Severe burn injury induces a prolonged hypermetabolic state that substantially reorganizes whole-body energy homeostasis [21]. Severe burn injury is followed by a sustained hypermetabolic response, mediated by elevated catecholamines, cortisol, and inflammatory cytokines, resulting in increased resting energy expenditure and prolonged catabolism [10]. Compared to other forms of critical illness, burn-induced hypermetabolism is more pronounced and can persist for years after injury [8, 22].

Clinically, this manifests as extreme elevations in resting energy expenditure, heightened protein catabolism, systemic insulin resistance, and persistent inflammation. This systemic derangement can last for months after trauma, creating a sustained mismatch between cellular energy requirements and metabolic substrate availability [7, 23–27]. Unlike the transient metabolic stress observed in many acute injuries, burn-induced hypermetabolism persists long after wound closure, imposing prolonged adaptive pressure on peripheral tissues.

Skeletal muscle is particularly exposed under these catabolic conditions. As the largest reservoir of protein in the body and a central regulator of metabolic flux, skeletal muscle occupies a pivotal position in burn-induced catabolic signaling [8]. Elevated levels of pro-inflammatory cytokines, glucocorticoids, and oxidative mediators favor proteolytic dominance and metabolic dysregulation [28]. These transitions do not simply reduce muscle mass; they disrupt proteostatic balance and increase the adaptive load required to sustain structural and metabolic integrity.

These alterations also occur against a backdrop of sustained energetic demand. Increased substrate cycling, futile metabolic loops, and ongoing inflammatory activation force muscle fibers to operate under chronically elevated metabolic pressure. When demand rises and substrate utilization is simultaneously impaired, skeletal muscle becomes increasingly dependent on continuous adaptation to maintain function. Failure of this adaptation contributes to the chronic weakness and delayed recovery frequently seen in burn survivors [29]. In this context, skeletal muscle functions not simply as a passive victim of systemic stress but as an active metabolic interface required to buffer prolonged energetic and inflammatory overload.

2.2 Mitochondrial vulnerability under stress

Mitochondria form the bioenergetic hub essential for muscle contraction and intracellular homeostasis. After burn trauma, substantial evidence demonstrates mitochondrial pathology, including altered cristae architecture, reduced oxidative phosphorylation (OXPHOS) efficiency, dysregulated reactive oxygen species (ROS) production, and therapeutic attempts targeting mitochondrial dynamics [30–32]. Severe burn trauma results in rapid reductions in skeletal muscle tissue pO_2 and increased mitochondrial ROS production within hours of injury [33].

Post-burn mitochondrial dysfunction may not manifest as a complete bioenergetic collapse under basal conditions. Instead, injured muscle often displays an erosion of functional reserve, whereby resting bioenergetic parameters appear relatively preserved, but the capacity to augment ATP production during metabolic or inflammatory challenges is impaired [34]. This erosion is reflected by reduced spare respiratory capacity and impaired stress-induced upregulation of oxidative phosphorylation. Under physiological load, bioenergetic machinery may remain active at rest yet fail to appropriately scale its output, rendering the system increasingly brittle under sustained stress.

Chronic oxidative stress further amplifies this vulnerability. Excessive ROS damages mitochondrial DNA, protein complexes, and membrane lipids, establishing a feedback cycle of progressive bioenergetic inefficiency [35, 36]. Imbalance in mitochondrial fission–fusion dynamics also impairs network remodeling in response to rising energetic demand [37]. Together, these changes leave mitochondria progressively unable to meet physiological demands.

Preservation of mitochondrial quality control, therefore, becomes essential: sustained adaptive capacity determines whether skeletal muscle can withstand the metabolic and inflammatory challenges imposed by severe burn injury.

2.3 Consequences for muscle performance and recovery

The functional implications of stress-induced mitochondrial vulnerability extend beyond cellular bioenergetics. Skeletal muscle relies on the capacity to scale ATP production during periods of increased demand, such as rehabilitation, infection, or ongoing inflammatory activation. When mitochondrial reserve capacity is reduced, even moderate additional stress may precipitate energetic insufficiency.

This impaired adaptability contributes to reduced stress tolerance at the tissue level. Burn patients frequently demonstrate prolonged weakness, decreased endurance, and delayed recovery despite apparent stabilization of systemic parameters [38]. Over time, recurrent episodes of metabolic overload without adequate restoration of homeostasis may promote structural remodeling and progressive muscle wasting. These observations suggest that skeletal muscle dysfunction after burn injury may be better understood as a failure of adaptive resilience rather than a simple deficit in baseline metabolic activity. Mitochondrial instability under stress provides a mechanistic foundation upon which disturbances in quality control and proteostasis can develop.

Skeletal muscle serves as a principal metabolic reservoir following burn injury, providing amino acids to support wound healing and acute-phase protein synthesis [39]. Burn-induced skeletal muscle dysfunction reflects not only the loss of contractile proteins but also impairments in mitochondrial content and function [39]. Mitochondrial dysfunction and dysregulated mitophagy are increasingly recognized as central mediators of burn pathology and wound healing [40]. Whether mitochondrial quality control pathways are sufficient to sustain adaptive capacity under chronic burn-induced stress remains unresolved, setting the stage for the examination of autophagy and mitophagy dynamics in the following chapter.

3 Autophagy and mitophagy in burn injury: Resolving apparent contradictions in the literature

3.1 Basal autophagy and mitophagy in skeletal muscle

Autophagy and mitophagy are fundamental pillars of skeletal muscle homeostasis [41]. Autophagy is more than a simple degradative pathway; it recycles substrates and sustains cellular adaptation under metabolic demand [42]. Disruption of autophagy results in impaired mitochondrial respiration and increased oxidative stress, linking autophagic deficiency directly to bioenergetic dysfunction [43].

Mitochondrial quality control operates through multi-tiered mechanisms, extending beyond mitophagy to include protein-level proteostasis, mitochondrial-derived vesicles, and coordinated biogenesis pathways [44].

The post-mitotic nature of myofibers and their high metabolic demand necessitate continuous organelle and protein turnover to preserve structural integrity and oxidative efficiency [45]. Circadian regulation and exercise timing further influence muscle regeneration and mitochondrial remodeling, highlighting that temporal coordination shapes adaptive capacity [46].

Under basal conditions, autophagy clears damaged proteins, while mitophagy selectively eliminates dysfunctional mitochondria to maintain oxidative capacity and limit reactive oxygen species production. Canonical pathways involving PINK1-Parkin signaling orchestrate mitochondrial recognition and elimination under stress [47].

Skeletal muscle exhibits relatively high constitutive autophagic activity compared to most other tissues [48]. This elevated turnover reflects ongoing mechanical load and fluctuating energy demand. Both defective and excessive autophagy can be detrimental, underscoring the importance of regulated flux rather than simplistic pathway activation or suppression [49].

Mitophagy is also dynamically induced during metabolic stress, such as exercise, in an AMPK-ULK1-dependent manner [50]. In this physiological context, autophagy and mitophagy are cytoprotective and tightly integrated into adaptive mitochondrial remodeling.

This picture becomes harder to interpret in pathological states, such as burn injury.

3.2 Reported findings post-burn injury: Apparent contradictions

Experimental studies evaluating autophagy and mitophagy after severe burn injuries have yielded heterogeneous findings.

Some report increased LC3-II levels, enhanced BNIP3 or Parkin expression, and elevated autophagosome formation, suggesting pathway activation [40, 51, 52]. In rodent models, increased LC3-II and Beclin-1 have been associated with muscle wasting, and pharmacologic autophagy inhibition partially attenuated atrophy [53].

Human muscle biopsies during the early flow phase demonstrate elevated proteolytic signaling without suppression of translational pathways, suggesting early atrophy is driven predominantly by increased degradation [54].

Direct evidence of mitochondrial dysfunction includes reduced ATP synthesis and downregulation of oxidative phosphorylation genes [30]. Burn injury also induces mitochondrial membrane potential loss and increased superoxide production, mediated partly by inflammatory DAMP signaling [55].

Burn impairs insulin-stimulated Akt/PKB activation and downstream p70S6K signaling, despite systemic hypermetabolism [56, 57]. The balance between synthesis and degradation is, therefore, disrupted [56].

Taken together, the literature describes:

(1) Increased autophagic markers

(2) Mitochondrial dysfunction

(3) Persistent oxidative stress

(4) Progressive muscle wasting

If autophagy is protective, why does its activation coexist with muscle atrophy? This apparent contradiction has led to ambiguity.

3.3 The core conceptual gap: Basal flux is not adaptive capacity

To borrow a metaphor from cardiology, evaluating autophagy solely under basal conditions is analogous to interpreting cardiac health from a resting electrocardiogram alone. Many patients with normal resting ECGs reveal latent pathology only during stress testing. A resting electrocardiogram cannot detect occult coronary ischemia, only a stress test can. Likewise, skeletal muscle may exhibit seemingly adequate (or increased) basal autophagic flux while failing to mount an appropriate mitophagy response under metabolic load.

Much of the earlier historical confusion stemmed from an overly reductive interpretation, in which autophagic marker abundance was taken as a direct measurement of pathway effectiveness. The field appropriately moved from static measurements to flux assessment [58, 59]. However, even flux assays are typically conducted under basal conditions [60]. Basal flux is a steady-state descriptor; adaptive responsiveness is a dynamic property.

An elevated basal autophagy rate may represent compensatory activation in response to upstream stress, rather than improved mitochondrial resilience. Conversely, reduced basal flux following therapeutic intervention may reflect alleviation of metabolic overload, rather than impaired autophagic machinery.

This distinction is exemplified in phosphodiesterase-5 inhibition studies on burn-induced muscle dysfunction. Burn injury increased basal autophagy flux, which decreased following treatment [60]. While superficially suggestive of autophagy suppression, the original interpretation emphasized that improved perfusion and reduced stress burden diminished the need for compensatory autophagic activation. Decreased basal flux in this setting reflected restored homeostasis, not impaired autophagy.

A similar ambiguity emerged in the trehalose debate. Trehalose has been described as an mTOR-independent autophagy inducer and TFEB activator [61]. Yet subsequent studies [62, 63] reported LC3-II and p62 accumulation, consistent with impaired flux under certain conditions. Even when flux was analyzed, trehalose seemed to block the basal autophagy flux. If trehalose restores stress-responsive mitophagy in disease states where this capacity is impaired, the observed reduction in basal flux need not indicate autophagy suppression. Rather, it may instead reflect a normalization of compensatory overactivation (a return toward homeostatic turnover rather than suppression). On this reading, the apparent contradiction dissolves. Yet trehalose reduces basal flux in healthy systems too, where no such overcompensation exists to resolve. If the same outcome arises by a different mechanism, basal flux alone cannot tell them apart, and the more important question may be what trehalose does to mitophagy when the system is actually under load.

Neither static nor basal flux measurements, however, assess stimulus-coupled mitophagy responsiveness under metabolic load. Without stress-challenge paradigms, both approaches remain incomplete.

3.4 Towards a stress-responsive framework

Severe burn injury imposes persistent metabolic and inflammatory stress [32, 55]. Under these conditions, mitochondrial quality control becomes a stress-responsive adaptive mechanism rather than a simple housekeeping turnover.

Mitochondrial reserve capacity (spare respiratory capacity) represents the bioenergetic buffer that determines stress tolerance [64]. Loss of reserve can occur despite preserved basal respiration [65, 66]. The decisive biological variable may not be basal autophagic flux but rather the ability of the system to scale mitophagy and maintain bioenergetic reserve under load.

What appears contradictory across burn studies may reflect differences in injury phase, stress intensity, or adaptive reserve capacity, rather than opposing biology.

Reconciling these observations requires separating steady-state turnover from adaptive response capacity.

This distinction reframes how therapeutic strategies aimed at restoring mitochondrial resilience in burn-induced skeletal muscle dysfunction should be evaluated.

4. Mitophagy response failure as a unifying concept

4.1 Limitations of static and basal flux-based assessments

Interpretation of autophagy and mitophagy in burn-injured skeletal muscle has traditionally relied on measurements of protein abundance or basal flux assays. Autophagy in skeletal muscle extends beyond basal housekeeping and includes stress adaptation and survival regulation [67]. Markers such as LC3 lipidation, p62/SQSTM1, BNIP3, NIX, and Parkin are frequently used as indicators of pathway engagement [58]. However, these approaches remain limited in their ability to assess functional mitochondrial quality control under physiologically relevant stress conditions. Persistent mitochondrial dysfunction has been repeatedly documented in burn-injured skeletal muscle.

A central conceptual problem lies in distinguishing basal turnover from adaptive capacity [68]. Basal flux reflects steady-state homeostasis but does not measure the ability of the system to scale mitochondrial clearance in response to metabolic or inflammatory stress. Dysregulated autophagy may manifest as either increased autophagosome formation or impaired lysosomal fusion, complicating the interpretation of static marker accumulation [69].

An additional analogy may be drawn from mechanical systems. Even a failing engine may appear to function normally at idle speed, yet stall when pushed toward its operational limits. Similarly, skeletal muscle mitochondria in diseases such as critical illnesses may maintain basal turnover while lacking sufficient reserve capacity to respond to sustained metabolic demand.

4.2 Stress-induced mitophagy and adaptive failure in burn injury

Instead of representing a steady-state disturbance, severe burn injury imposes a sustained metabolic and inflammatory stressor [8]. In contrast to physiological stress models, such as exercise, where stress-induced mitophagy is tightly coupled to mitochondrial biogenesis and improved organelle quality [70, 71], burn injury may be characterized by the failure of stimulus-coupled mitochondrial clearance.

Mechanistically, stress-induced mitophagy failure may arise at three interconnected levels:

(1) Initiation-completion uncoupling: Upstream activation of autophagy signaling does not guarantee effective organelle clearance under high demand [50, 72].

(2) Lysosomal insufficiency: Metabolic overload and oxidative stress may impair lysosomal acidification and autophagosome–lysosome fusion, resulting in apparent pathway activation without functional clearance [73, 74].

(3) Organelle-cytoskeletal integration defects: Disruption of vesicular trafficking and tubulin-VDAC coupling may compromise mitochondrial permeability and bioenergetic stability [75].

Under such conditions, preserved basal mitophagy flux may mask impaired adaptive capacity. As in heart failure, where resting cardiac output may be maintained despite exercise intolerance [76], skeletal muscle mitochondria may appear stable at baseline while harboring diminished reserve (**Figure 1**). Mitochondrial networks approaching criticality become susceptible to synchronized energetic collapse under minor perturbations [77].

4.3 Mechanistic basis and functional consequences of mitophagy response failure

Mitophagy response impairment means more than reduced pathway activity; it reflects an inability to appropriately augment mitochondrial clearance in proportion to stress intensity. In skeletal muscle, this stress-responsive scaling is mediated through convergent signaling pathways, including AMPK–ULK1 activation and receptor-mediated mechanisms beyond canonical PINK1–Parkin signaling [50, 78, 79]. Under physiological stress, such as exercise, mitophagy is

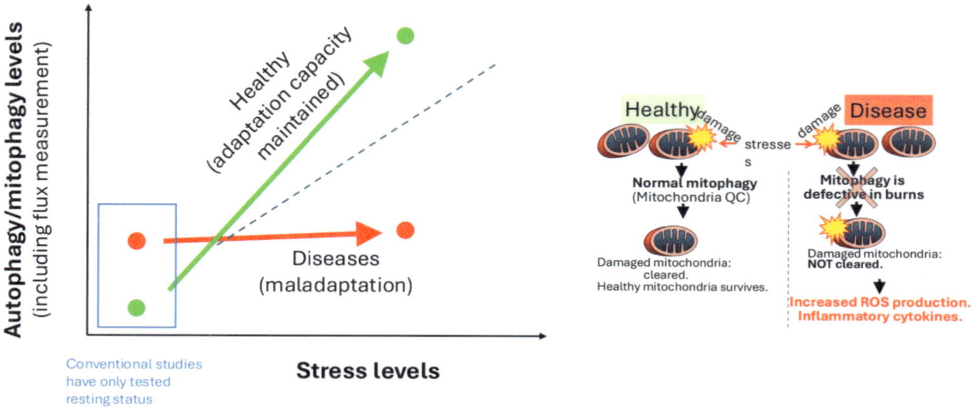

Figure 1.
Basal autophagy markers do not reflect stress-responsive mitophagy capacity. Conventional assessments (left panel) quantify basal marker abundance or flux under resting conditions, often leading to conflicting interpretations regarding pathway activation or suppression. These measurements are frequently equated with functional autophagic efficiency. However, skeletal muscle survival under burn injury depends primarily on the ability to scale mitophagy in response to metabolic or inflammatory stress (including elevated levels of inflammatory cytokines, endotoxins due to gut permeability alterations and altered microbiomes, and/or tissue hypoxia (including failure in oxygen utility). Burn injury may preserve or even elevate basal turnover while impairing stimulus-coupled mitophagy responsiveness, resulting in mitochondrial reserve collapse despite apparent pathway activation. Such mismatching between supply-demand relationship for mitophagy can result in the poor clearance of dysfunctional mitochondria.

tightly coordinated with mitochondrial biogenesis, allowing adaptive remodeling and preservation of organelle quality [70, 80].

In burn injury, however, this adaptive scaling may become uncoupled. Mechanistically, the failure of stress-induced mitophagy can arise at multiple levels. Upstream signaling activation does not guarantee effective organelle clearance under sustained metabolic load [50]. Mitophagy initiation and completion require coordinated kinase activation and lysosomal competence [78]. Persistent oxidative stress and inflammatory signaling may impair lysosomal acidification and autophagosome–lysosome fusion, resulting in apparent pathway activation without functional clearance [73, 74]. In parallel, the disruption of cytoskeletal organization and tubulin–VDAC interactions may compromise mitochondrial permeability regulation and substrate flux, further destabilizing bioenergetic homeostasis [75].

Mitochondrial quality control (MQC) integrates fission, fusion, mitophagy, and biogenesis into a coordinated adaptive network [44, 81]. Mitochondria function not only as bioenergetic units but also as signaling platforms responsive to calcium flux, redox status, and metabolite-derived second messengers [82–85]. When stress-responsive clearance is impaired, dysfunctional mitochondria accumulate within this network, destabilizing its adaptive architecture.

The consequence of an impaired mitophagy response is the erosion of mitochondrial reserve capacity. Loss of spare respiratory capacity renders muscle fibers unable to meet ATP demand during metabolic or inflammatory challenges, even when basal respiration appears preserved [64–66]. Mitochondrial networks approaching a state of criticality become increasingly susceptible to synchronized depolarization and energetic collapse under minor perturbations [77].

Preserved basal mitophagy flux may, therefore, mask diminished adaptive reserve, analogous to maintained resting cardiac output in heart failure despite exercise intolerance [76].

Over repeated stress episodes, insufficient restoration of mitochondrial homeostasis promotes oxidative stress amplification, proteostatic imbalance, and dysregulated anabolic signaling [28, 86, 87]. Disruption of fusion–fission balance, including MFN2- and DRP1-mediated dynamics, further impairs segregation and removal of damaged organelles [88–90]. A similar dissociation between preserved basal turnover and impaired stress-induced mitophagy has been demonstrated in aging skeletal muscle [15, 76].

Mitophagy response failure ultimately constrains muscle regenerative capacity. Efficient repair requires coordinated mitochondrial remodeling and renewal in differentiating satellite cells [3, 91]. Persistent mitochondrial fragility generates a pro-oxidative and inflammatory environment that limits structural recovery and can promote progressive functional decline [92].

Skeletal muscle wasting after severe burn injury may reflect a progressive loss of stress tolerance capacity rather than a static dysregulation of autophagy pathways. Burn-associated pathology may emerge not from absolute suppression or hyperactivation of mitophagy but from an impaired ability to execute mitochondrial quality control dynamically under sustained stress.

5. Why mitophagy response failure persists: A bidirectional neuroimmune–muscle amplification network

The mitophagy response failure described in Chap. 4 raises a central unresolved question: why might this defect persist and progressively amplify in some patients under the sustained systemic stress conditions that follow severe burn injury?

While earlier sections focused primarily on intracellular mechanisms of mitochondrial quality control, skeletal muscle does not operate in isolation. Severe burn injury imposes a prolonged neuroimmune and metabolic stress environment, in which skeletal muscle both responds to and actively shapes systemic signaling. In this context, mitophagy dysregulation is best understood not solely as a cell-intrinsic defect but as the product of an interaction between intrinsic mitochondrial vulnerability and persistent extrinsic stress load.

We propose that burn-associated skeletal muscle dysfunction is maintained through a bidirectional amplification network linking mitochondrial stress signaling, neuroimmune activation, and systemic metabolic dysregulation. Impaired stress-responsive mitophagy represents an intrinsic vulnerability that limits adaptive mitochondrial quality control, whereas sustained neuroimmune activation functions as a chronic extrinsic load that continuously challenges this capacity and stabilizes maladaptive responses.

5.1 Conceptual framework: Intrinsic vulnerability meets extrinsic load

Under physiological conditions, mitochondrial stress is managed through coordinated quality control mechanisms, including mitophagy, biogenesis, and redox buffering. In severe burn injury, however, persistent metabolic and inflammatory stress places sustained demands on skeletal muscle mitochondria.

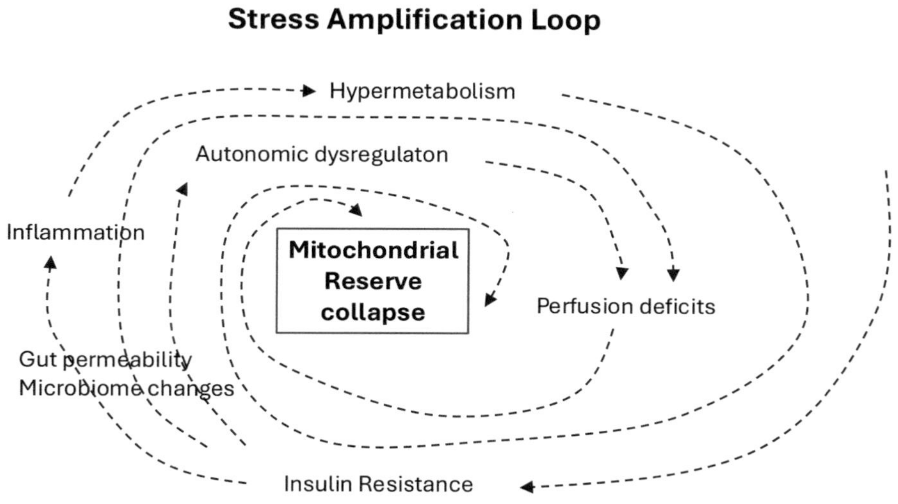

Figure 2.
Stress amplification loop driving mitophagy response failure after severe burn injury. Severe burn injury generates persistent hypermetabolic and inflammatory stress that disrupts mitochondrial reserve capacity and challenges mitochondrial quality control in skeletal muscle. Systemic inflammation, autonomic dysregulation, insulin resistance, and perfusion deficits collectively increase mitochondrial workload and oxidative burden. Although basal autophagy may be preserved or elevated, insufficient stress-responsive mitophagy permits the accumulation of dysfunctional mitochondria during periods of high metabolic demand. These organelles amplify reactive oxygen species generation and release mtDAMPs, further intensifying systemic inflammation and metabolic instability, thereby forming a self-reinforcing amplification loop. The model integrates intrinsic adaptive insufficiency (impaired stress-responsive mitophagy and reduced reserve capacity) with persistent extrinsic load (neuroimmune-driven hypermetabolism) to explain how mitochondrial stress becomes chronic rather than resolving adaptively. This progressive mismatch between demand and adaptive capacity may only become apparent under sustained or repeated stress, thereby explaining why mitochondrial dysfunction can remain latent at rest but manifest during metabolic challenge.

When stress-responsive mitophagy capacity is insufficient relative to systemic load, dysfunctional mitochondria accumulate and progressively destabilize cellular homeostasis.

This interaction may be conceptualized as the convergence of two forces:

(1) Intrinsic vulnerability: impaired stress-responsive mitophagy and reduced mitochondrial reserve capacity

(2) Extrinsic load: sustained neuroimmune-driven hypermetabolism and inflammatory signaling

Rather than representing independent processes, these components interact dynamically. Extrinsic stress increases mitochondrial workload, while intrinsic adaptive failure amplifies inflammatory signaling and metabolic instability, reinforcing systemic stress (**Figure 2**).

5.2 Neuroimmune activation as a source of persistent extrinsic load

Severe burn injury induces sustained neuroimmune activation characterized by central inflammatory signaling, autonomic dysregulation, and endocrine stress responses. Peripheral cytokines such as IL-1β, TNF-α, and IL-6 propagate neuroinflammatory responses through both humoral and neural pathways and can disrupt blood–brain barrier integrity [93]. Immune-to-brain communication occurs via parallel neural and humoral pathways, including vagal afferents and cytokine signaling at circumventricular organs [94]. Experimental models demonstrate rapid upregulation of TNF-α, IL-1β, and ICAM-1 expression within the brain following cutaneous burn injury [95].

Neuroimmune activation subsequently modulates:

(i) Sympathetic nervous system activity

(ii) Hypothalamic–pituitary–adrenal axis tone

(iii) Endocrine stress signaling

(iv) Systemic energy expenditure

Sustained sympathetic activation increases basal metabolic rate, lipolysis, and skeletal muscle substrate flux. Propranolol-mediated β-adrenergic blockade attenuates resting energy expenditure and reverses muscle-protein catabolism in severely burned children, underscoring the central role of catecholamine-driven hypermetabolism [96]. Urinary cortisol and catecholamine excretion remain elevated for weeks to months after severe burn injury [97].

These centrally mediated mechanisms do not necessarily directly injure mitochondria. Rather, they increase the metabolic and inflammatory load under which mitochondrial quality control systems must operate. Neuroimmune-driven hypermetabolism does not directly initiate mitochondrial injury; rather, it functions as a sustained physiological stress test that increases metabolic demand and oxidative burden, thereby revealing whether mitochondrial quality control systems, including stress-responsive mitophagy, can scale appropriately. When this adaptive capacity is insufficient, dysfunctional mitochondria accumulate, and mitochondrial reserve capacity declines, leading to progressive energetic instability under continued stress.

Muscles with preserved adaptive capacity may tolerate such a load. When stress-responsive mitophagy capacity is limited, however, sustained neuroimmune drive may precipitate failure. This failure is not necessarily immediate but can emerge progressively as repeated or sustained metabolic challenges exhaust mitochondrial reserve capacity over time, eventually shifting the system from a compensated to a decompensated state.

This stress load operates across multiple functional layers, affecting not only mitophagy regulation but also progressively eroding mitochondrial reserve capacity, thereby linking defects in quality control to downstream energetic insufficiency.

5.3 Retrograde signaling from muscle to systemic networks

Communication between skeletal muscle and systemic regulatory networks operates in both directions. Beyond autonomic and endocrine inputs, skeletal muscle actively contributes to systemic signaling through mitochondrial stress responses, the release of mtDAMPs, and the secretion of stress-responsive myokines such as FGF21 and GDF15.

Altered muscle metabolic states influence neuronal activity and plasticity via metabolite-sensitive and activity-dependent signaling pathways [98]. Burn injury induces microglial activation, spinal inflammatory signaling, motor neuron loss, and skeletal muscle wasting, with attenuation observed through α7AChR-mediated modulation of microglial tone [99].

Mitochondrial stress within muscle activates the integrated stress response, inducing the secretion of stress-responsive cytokines, as noted above, which exert systemic metabolic and neuroendocrine effects [100]. Mitochondrial stress can also induce the cytosolic release of mtDNA via VDAC oligomerization-dependent macropores, activating cGAS–STING signaling [101].

Within this bidirectional network, stress-responsive mitophagy functions as a nodal checkpoint. When mitochondrial clearance scales appropriately with stress, perturbations resolve. When clearance capacity is insufficient, dysfunctional mitochondria accumulate, inflammatory signaling amplifies, and the network stabilizes in a high-stress state. Mitophagy may critically influence whether transient injury signals dissipate or escalate into self-sustaining amplification.

5.4 A self-reinforcing amplification loop

This perspective does not imply a uniform, progressive deterioration across all patients. Clinical trajectories after burn injury are heterogeneous, with many individuals demonstrating gradual recovery, while a subset exhibits prolonged or maladaptive responses.

Burn-injured skeletal muscle may exhibit reduced adaptive capacity despite appearing metabolically adequate at rest. Hypermetabolic and hyperinflammatory responses persist for up to three years after burn injury, sustaining the extrinsic load on mitochondrial quality control systems [7].

The interaction can be conceptualized as:

Intrinsic vulnerability (impaired stress-responsive mitophagy capacity)

+

Extrinsic load (neuroimmune-driven hypermetabolism and inflammatory tone)

→ Failure of mitochondrial turnover under demand

When damaged mitochondria are not efficiently cleared during high metabolic flux, ATP production declines while ROS generation increases. Elevated ROS further damages mitochondrial proteins and DNA, reinforcing mitochondrial dysfunction. Mitochondrial fragmentation can trigger sterile inflammation through TLR9-dependent DNA-sensing pathways, promoting IL-6 responses, muscle atrophy, and reduced physical performance [102].

Over time, this interaction may stabilize in a subset of patients into a maladaptive steady state characterized by sustained hypermetabolism, impaired mitochondrial renewal, and progressive muscle wasting. Burn injury can sustain hypermetabolism and skeletal muscle dysfunction long after wound closure, reinforcing a prolonged systemic load [8].

This systems-level model does not require exclusive causality from either the muscle or the CNS. Burn injury initiates a distributed perturbation in which intrinsic adaptive insufficiency and extrinsic stress signaling dynamically reinforce one another. Impaired stress-responsive mitophagy may function as a key bottleneck: when clearance scales with demand, mitochondrial stress resolves; when it fails, both local and systemic amplification follow [40].

If pathological progression is driven by an amplification loop, effective interventions may need to operate at multiple levels, either by reducing upstream systemic stress load, restoring stress-responsive mitochondrial quality control capacity, or both. The following chapter examines how emerging therapeutic strategies may be evaluated not only by their effects on basal pathway activity alone but also by their ability to restore adaptive mitochondrial resilience under stress.

6. Therapeutic implications: Restoring stress-responsive mitochondrial capacity

Therapeutic strategies for burn-induced skeletal muscle dysfunction have traditionally focused on suppressing inflammation or attenuating hypermetabolism. However, the framework developed in the preceding chapters suggests that the central pathological feature is not simply pathway overactivation or suppression, but rather impaired stress-responsive mitochondrial quality control under sustained systemic load. The decisive variable may be less about basal autophagic flux and more about adaptive mitophagy responsiveness and the preservation of mitochondrial reserve capacity during metabolic challenge. Therapeutic evaluation should, accordingly, move beyond static measurements of pathway activation and instead determine whether interventions restore the ability of skeletal muscle mitochondria to scale appropriately in response to stress.

Within this model, therapeutic strategies can be organized along three complementary axes: reduction of upstream systemic stress load, restoration of stress-responsive mitochondrial quality control, and preservation of bioenergetic reserve capacity under sustained demand.

6.1 Reducing upstream stress burden: Restoring homeostatic balance

Severe burn injury imposes persistent hypermetabolic demand, inflammatory signaling, and impaired perfusion [26]. These upstream stressors elevate basal autophagic turnover as a compensatory mechanism.

In this context, interventions that reduce metabolic overload may normalize basal autophagy without directly targeting the autophagic machinery itself.

Phosphodiesterase-5 inhibition provides an instructive example. In burn-induced muscle atrophy, elevated basal autophagy flux was reduced following treatment [60]. Rather than indicating suppression of mitochondrial quality control, this likely reflected alleviation of perfusion deficits and reduced energetic stress, thereby diminishing the requirement for compensatory activation.

Reduced basal flux in this setting may represent restored equilibrium rather than impaired autophagy.

Optimizing insulin sensitivity, improving substrate delivery, and attenuating excessive catabolic signaling may similarly decrease mitochondrial stress burden and preserve reserve capacity [56, 65].

One therapeutic axis, therefore, involves reducing overload to restore the physiological set point of mitochondrial turnover.

DOI: http://dx.doi.org/10.5772/intechopen.1015862

6.2 Enhancing coordinated mitophagy responsiveness

A second therapeutic axis involves improving stimulus-coupled mitochondrial quality control.

Agents such as SGLT2 inhibitors have been associated with improved mitochondrial function and enhanced autophagy-related signaling in cardiac and skeletal muscle systems. Trehalose has been widely described as an mTOR-independent autophagy inducer and TFEB activator. GLP-1 receptor agonists and ivermectin have also been reported to modulate autophagy-associated pathways in various disease contexts. CoQ10 has demonstrated partial restoration of mitochondrial structure and insulin signaling in burn models [103–105].

However, the interpretation of these findings requires caution.

Increased LC3-II accumulation or altered flux under basal conditions does not automatically imply enhanced adaptive mitophagy responsiveness. As discussed in Chap. 3, marker changes observed at rest may reflect altered kinetics rather than improved stress resilience.

The critical question is not whether a compound "activates autophagy," but whether it restores the ability of skeletal muscle mitochondria to maintain spare respiratory capacity and coordinate degradation with biogenesis under load.

Agents that enhance lysosomal efficiency, support mitochondrial dynamics, improve redox buffering, or activate TFEB-mediated transcriptional programs may strengthen the adaptive capacity without necessarily increasing basal marker abundance.

Pharmacologic screening strategies should, therefore, incorporate stress-challenge paradigms rather than relying exclusively on resting flux measurements.

6.3 Neuroimmune modulation as a regulator of mitochondrial resilience

Skeletal muscle mitochondrial function exists within a broader neuroimmune regulatory network. Chronic inflammatory signaling and dysregulated autonomic tone may amplify mitochondrial stress in burn injuries.

While direct evidence linking neuroimmune-targeted therapies to improved mitophagy responsiveness remains limited, restoring equilibrium in systemic stress signaling may indirectly preserve mitochondrial reserve capacity.

Therapeutic strategies that dampen excessive inflammatory signaling may, therefore, synergize with metabolic and mitochondrial-targeted approaches.

6.4 Phase-sensitive and integrated therapeutic strategies

Burn injury evolves through acute, subacute, and chronic phases, each characterized by distinct metabolic and inflammatory phenotypes.

Early interventions may prioritize stabilization of systemic stress and prevention of mitochondrial overload. Later stages may benefit from interventions that promote remodeling and regenerative adaptation.

An integrated strategy combining:

(1) Reduction of upstream metabolic overload

(2) Restoration of stimulus-coupled mitophagy responsiveness

(3) Preservation of mitochondrial reserve capacity

(4) Neuroimmune stabilization

may offer a more coherent therapeutic approach than targeting isolated molecular markers.

Meaningful therapeutic endpoints should, therefore, include stress tolerance, recovery kinetics, and maintenance of spare respiratory capacity rather than static changes in LC3-II abundance alone.

Therapeutic success in burn-associated muscle dysfunction will, therefore, depend less on correcting isolated molecular abnormalities and more on restoring the capacity of mitochondria to respond adaptively under physiological stress.

7. Future directions and outstanding questions

Despite increasing awareness of mitochondrial dysfunction in burn-associated skeletal muscle pathophysiology, several key questions remain unresolved. A key challenge lies in devising experimental paradigms that quantitatively assess stress-responsive mitochondrial quality control processes in vivo rather than relying solely on resting state assessments. Traditional static measurements and basal flux assays are likely inadequate to detect adaptive capacity in physiologically relevant settings. Incorporating metabolic or inflammatory challenge protocols into experimental designs would enable mitophagy responsiveness to be assessed under conditions that more closely reflect the pathophysiological context of burn injury.

A further priority is understanding how mitochondrial quality control capacity shifts across the acute, subacute, and chronic phases of burn injury. When stress-responsive mitophagy becomes insufficient, and whether that capacity can be restored, are questions with direct implications for the timing of therapeutic intervention. Closely related is the need to clarify how neuroimmune activation interfaces with mitochondrial stress signaling. Mounting evidence supports bidirectional crosstalk between central inflammatory responses and peripheral metabolic regulation, but the mechanistic connections to mitochondrial homeostasis in skeletal muscle remain poorly defined.

In translational efforts, stress tolerance, recovery kinetics, and muscle performance under sustained demand should be measured alongside molecular marker normalization. Outcomes defined this way are more likely to capture the adaptive resilience that ultimately determines patient recovery.

8. Conclusions

Although autophagy and mitophagy are studied extensively in this context, interpreting findings has been muddied with inconsistencies. This chapter argues that the disconnect underlying much of this apparent contradiction may arise from an inability to separate basal pathway activity from adaptive stress responsiveness.

This reframing reconciles metabolic vulnerability, mitochondrial dysfunction, and neuroimmune dysregulation within a single model. Rather than a simple up- or downregulation of autophagy, burn-associated muscle pathology is better understood as a failure of adaptive capacity under prolonged stress, one that cannot be reduced to a fixed defect in any single pathway.

Therapeutic strategies targeting mitochondrial resilience through metabolic support, stress signaling modulation, and maintenance of quality control responsiveness may ultimately improve long-term functional recovery in burn survivors.

Conflict of Interest

Dr. Yasuhara has received lecture honoraria from Tokyo Central Beauty Clinic and has a research grant under review with the same institution. Dr. Tamura is currently affiliated with Tokyo Central Beauty Clinic. The authors declare that these relationships did not influence the content of this work.

Author details

Shingo E. Yasuhara[1,2]*, Zerong You[1], Diroji Antony[1,2] and Takahiko Tamura[1,3,4]

1 Department of Anesthesia, Critical Care and Pain Medicine, Massachusetts General Hospital and Harvard Medical School, Boston, USA

2 Shriners Hospitals for Children, Boston, USA

3 Tokyo Chuo Beauty Clinic, Osaka, Japan

4 Kochi University, Medical School, Kochi, Japan

*Address all correspondence to: syasuhara@mgh.harvard.edu

References

[1] Jeschke MG, van Baar ME, Choudhry MA, Chung KK, Gibran NS, Logsetty S. Burn injury. Nature Reviews Disease Primers. 2020;**6**(1):11

[2] Porter C, Tompkins RG, Finnerty CC, Sidossis LS, Suman OE, Herndon DN. The metabolic stress response to burn trauma: Current understanding and therapies. Lancet. 2016;**388**(10052):1417–1426

[3] Clark AT, Song J, Yao X, et al. Muscle homeostasis is disrupted in burned adults. Journal of Burn Care & Research 2019;**41**:33–40

[4] St-Pierre DMM, Choinière M, Forget R, Garrel DR. Muscle strength in individuals with healed burns. Archives of Physical Medicine and Rehabilitation. 1998;**79**(2):155–161

[5] Bonaldo P, Sandri M. Cellular and molecular mechanisms of muscle atrophy. Disease Models & Mechanisms. 2013;**6**(1):25–39

[6] Dombrecht D, Van Daele U, Van Asbroeck B, et al. Molecular mechanisms of post-burn muscle wasting and the therapeutic potential of physical exercise. Journal of Cachexia, Sarcopenia and Muscle 2023;**14**:758–770

[7] Jeschke MG, Gauglitz GG, Kulp GA, et al. Long-term persistance of the pathophysiologic response to severe burn injury. PLOS ONE 2011;**6**:e21245

[8] Knuth CM, Auger C, Jeschke MG. Burn-induced hypermetabolism and skeletal muscle dysfunction. American Journal of Physiology-Cell Physiology. 2021;**321**(1):C58–c71

[9] Song J, Clark A, Wade CE, Wolf SE. Skeletal muscle wasting after a severe burn is a consequence of cachexia and sarcopenia. Journal of Parenteral and Enteral Nutrition. 2021;**45**(8):1627–1633

[10] Williams FN, Herndon DN, Jeschke MG. The hypermetabolic response to burn injury and interventions to modify this response. Clinics in Plastic Surgery. 2009;**36**(4):583–596

[11] Polychronopoulou E, Herndon DN, Porter C. The Long-Term Impact of Severe Burn Trauma on Musculoskeletal Health. Journal of Burn Care & Research. 2018;**39**(6):869–880

[12] Chandel NS. Mitochondria as signaling organelles. BMC Biology. 2014;**12**:34

[13] D'Arcy MS. Mitophagy in health and disease. Molecular mechanisms, regulatory pathways, and therapeutic implications. Apoptosis. 2024;**29**(9-10):1415–1428

[14] Doblado L, Lueck C, Rey C, et al. Mitophagy in Human Diseases. International Journal of Molecular Sciences 2021;**22**:3903

[15] Picca A, Faitg J, Auwerx J, Ferrucci L, D'Amico D. Mitophagy in human health, ageing and disease. Nature Metabolism. 2023;**5**(12):2047–2061

[16] Zhu CL, Yao RQ, Li LX, et al. Mechanism of Mitophagy and Its Role in Sepsis Induced Organ Dysfunction: A Review. Frontiers in Cell and Developmental Biology. 2021;**9**:664896

[17] Prabhakaran HS, Hu D, He W, Luo G, Liou YC. Mitochondrial

dysfunction and mitophagy: Crucial players in burn trauma and wound healing. Burns & Trauma. 2023;**11**: tkad029

[18] Klawitter F, Ehler J, Bajorat R, Patejdl R. Mitochondrial Dysfunction in Intensive Care Unit-Acquired Weakness and Critical Illness Myopathy: A Narrative Review. International Journal of Molecular Sciences. 2023;**24**(6):5516

[19] Hu D, Sheeja Prabhakaran H, Zhang YY, Luo G, He W, Liou YC. Mitochondrial dysfunction in sepsis: Mechanisms and therapeutic perspectives. Critical Care. 2024;**28** (1):292

[20] Manoli I, Alesci S, Blackman MR, Su YA, Rennert OM, Chrousos GP. Mitochondria as key components of the stress response. Trends in Endocrinology & Metabolism. 2007;**18** (5):190–198

[21] Gauglitz GG, Herndon DN, Jeschke MG. Insulin resistance postburn: Underlying mechanisms and current therapeutic strategies. Journal of Burn Care & Research. 2008;**29** (5):683–694

[22] Osborne T, Wall B, Edgar DW, Fairchild T, Wood F. Current understanding of the chronic stress response to burn injury from human studies. Burns & Trauma. 2023;**11**: tkad007

[23] Gauglitz GG, Herndon DN, Kulp GA, Meyer III WJ, Jeschke MG. Abnormal Insulin Sensitivity Persists up to Three Years in Pediatric Patients Post-Burn. The Journal of Clinical Endocrinology & Metabolism. 2009;**94** (5):1656–1664

[24] Cree MG, Wolfe RR. Postburn trauma insulin resistance and fat metabolism. American Journal of Physiology-Endocrinology and Metabolism. 2008;**294**(1):E1–E9

[25] Cree MG, Fram RY, Barr D, Chinkes DL, Wolfe RR, Herndon DN. Insulin resistance, secretion and breakdown are increased 9 months following severe burn injury. Burns: Journal of the International Society for Burn Injuries. 2009;**35**(1):63–69

[26] Porter C, Herndon DN, Børsheim E, et al. Long-Term Skeletal Muscle Mitochondrial Dysfunction is Associated with Hypermetabolism in Severely Burned Children. Journal of Burn Care & Research 2016;**37**:53–63

[27] Mulder PPG, Vlig M, Boekema B, et al. Persistent Systemic Inflammation in Patients With Severe Burn Injury Is Accompanied by Influx of Immature Neutrophils and Shifts in T Cell Subsets and Cytokine Profiles. Frontiers in Immunology. 2021;**11**:621222

[28] Fang CH, Li BG, Fischer DR, et al. Burn injury upregulates the activity and gene expression of the 20 S proteasome in rat skeletal muscle. Clinical Science (London) 2000;**99**:181–187

[29] Smith RL, Soeters MR, Wüst RCI, Houtkooper RH. Metabolic Flexibility as an Adaptation to Energy Resources and Requirements in Health and Disease. Endocrine Reviews. 2018;**39**(4):489–517

[30] Padfield KE, Astrakas LG, Zhang Q, et al. Burn injury causes mitochondrial dysfunction in skeletal muscle. Proceedings of the National Academy of Sciences of the United States of America 2005;**102**:5368–5373

[31] Chao T, Gómez BI, Heard TC, Smith BW, Dubick MA, Burmeister DM. Burn-induced reductions in mitochondrial abundance and efficiency are more pronounced with small volumes of colloids in swine. American Journal of Physiology-Cell Physiology. 2019;**317**(6):C1229–C1238

[32] Nakazawa H, Ikeda K, Shinozaki S, et al. Burn-induced muscle metabolic derangements and mitochondrial dysfunction are associated with activation of HIF-1α and mTORC1: Role of protein farnesylation. Scientific Reports 2017;**7**:6618

[33] Khan N, Mupparaju SP, Mintzopoulos D, et al. Burn trauma in skeletal muscle results in oxidative stress as assessed by in vivo electron paramagnetic resonance. Molecular Medicine Reports 2008;**1**:813–819

[34] Hill BG, Dranka BP, Zou L, Chatham JC, Darley-Usmar VM. Importance of the bioenergetic reserve capacity in response to cardiomyocyte stress induced by 4-hydroxynonenal. The Biochemical Journal. 2009;**424**(1):99–107

[35] Olsen RK, Cornelius N, Gregersen N. Redox signalling and mitochondrial stress responses; lessons from inborn errors of metabolism. Journal of Inherited Metabolic Disease. 2015;**38**(4):703–719

[36] Porter C, Herndon DN, Børsheim E, et al. Uncoupled skeletal muscle mitochondria contribute to hypermetabolism in severely burned adults. American Journal of Physiology-Endocrinology and Metabolism 2014;**307**:E462–467

[37] Eisner V, Picard M, Hajnóczky G. Mitochondrial dynamics in adaptive and maladaptive cellular stress responses. Nature Cell Biology. 2018;**20**(7):755–765

[38] Grisbrook TL, Elliott CM, Edgar DW, Wallman KE, Wood FM, Reid SL. Burn-injured adults with long term functional impairments demonstrate the same response to resistance training as uninjured controls. Burns. 2013;**39**(4):680–686

[39] Porter C, Herndon DN, Sidossis LS, Børsheim E. The impact of severe burns on skeletal muscle mitochondrial function. Burns. 2013;**39**(6):1039–1047

[40] Prabhakaran HS, Hu D, He W, Luo G, Liou Y-C. Mitochondrial dysfunction and mitophagy: Crucial players in burn trauma and wound healing. Burns & Trauma. 2023;**11**: tkad021

[41] Masiero E, Agatea L, Mammucari C, et al. Autophagy Is Required to Maintain Muscle Mass. Cell Metabolism 2009;**10**:507–515

[42] Mizushima N, Komatsu M. Autophagy: Renovation of cells and tissues. Cell. 2011;**147**(4):728–741

[43] Wu JJ, Quijano C, Chen E, et al. Mitochondrial dysfunction and oxidative stress mediate the physiological impairment induced by the disruption of autophagy. Aging (Albany NY) 2009;**1**:425–437

[44] Pickles S, Vigié P, Youle RJ. Mitophagy and Quality Control Mechanisms in Mitochondrial Maintenance. Current Biology. 2018;**28**(4):R170–r185

[45] Wagers AJ, Conboy IM. Cellular and Molecular Signatures of Muscle

Regeneration: Current Concepts and Controversies in Adult Myogenesis. Cell. 2005;**122**(5):659–667

[46] Su Z, Xiang L. Exercise, circadian rhythms, and muscle regeneration: A path to healthy aging. Frontiers in Neuroscience. 2025;**19**:1633835

[47] Youle RJ, Narendra DP. Mechanisms of mitophagy. Nature Reviews Molecular Cell Biology. 2011;**12**(1):9–14

[48] Neel BA, Lin Y, Pessin JE. Skeletal muscle autophagy: A new metabolic regulator. Trends in Endocrinology & Metabolism. 2013;**24**(12):635–643

[49] Grumati P, Bonaldo P. Autophagy in Skeletal Muscle Homeostasis and in Muscular Dystrophies. Cells. 2012;**1**(3):325–345

[50] Laker RC, Drake JC, Wilson RJ, et al. Ampk phosphorylation of Ulk1 is required for targeting of mitochondria to lysosomes in exercise-induced mitophagy. Nature Communications 2017;**8**:548

[51] Yu Y, Yang L, Han S, et al. MIR-190B Alleviates Cell Autophagy and Burn-Induced Skeletal Muscle Wasting via Modulating PHLPP1/Akt/FoxO3A Signaling Pathway. Shock 2019;**52**:513–521

[52] Song J, Chowdhury IH, Choudhuri S, et al. Acute muscle mass loss was alleviated with HMGB1 neutralizing antibody treatment in severe burned rats. Scientific Reports 2023;**13**:10250

[53] Zhao F, Yu Y, Liu W, et al. Small Molecular Weight Soybean Protein-Derived Peptides Nutriment Attenuates Rat Burn Injury-Induced Muscle Atrophy by Modulation of Ubiquitin-Proteasome System and Autophagy Signaling Pathway. Journal of Agricultural and Food Chemistry 2018;**66**:2724–2734

[54] Merritt EK, Cross JM, Bamman MM. Inflammatory and protein metabolism signaling responses in human skeletal muscle after burn injury. Journal of Burn Care & Research. 2012;**33**(2):291–297

[55] Ueki R, Liu L, Kashiwagi S, et al. Role of Elevated Fibrinogen in Burn-Induced Mitochondrial Dysfunction: Protective Effects of Glycyrrhizin. Shock 2016;**46**:382–389

[56] Sugita H, Kaneki M, Sugita M, Yasukawa T, Yasuhara S, Martyn JA. Burn injury impairs insulin-stimulated Akt/PKB activation in skeletal muscle. American Journal of Physiology-Endocrinology and Metabolism. 2005;**288**(3):E585–591

[57] Gao S, Zhao X, Leng Y, Xia Z. Dietary supplementation with inulin improves burn-induced skeletal muscle atrophy by regulating gut microbiota disorders. Scientific Reports. 2024;**14**(1):2328

[58] Ju JS, Varadhachary AS, Miller SE, Weihl CC. Quantitation of "autophagic flux" in mature skeletal muscle. Autophagy. 2010;**6**(7):929–935

[59] Yoshii SR, Mizushima N. Monitoring and Measuring Autophagy. International Journal of Molecular Sciences. 2017;**18**(9):1865

[60] Hosokawa S, Koseki H, Nagashima M, et al. Title efficacy of phosphodiesterase 5 inhibitor on distant burn-induced muscle autophagy,

microcirculation, and survival rate. American Journal of Physiology-Endocrinology and Metabolism 2013;**304**:E922–933

[61] Sharma J, di Ronza A, Lotfi P, Sardiello M. Lysosomes and Brain Health. Annual Review of Neuroscience. 2018;**41**:255–276

[62] Yoon YS, Cho ED, Jung Ahn W, Won Lee K, Lee SJ, Lee HJ. Is trehalose an autophagic inducer? Unraveling the roles of non-reducing disaccharides on autophagic flux and alpha-synuclein aggregation. Cell Death & Disease. 2017;**8**(10):e3091

[63] Lee H-J, Yoon Y-S, Lee S-J. Mechanism of neuroprotection by trehalose: Controversy surrounding autophagy induction. Cell Death & Disease. 2018;**9**(7):712

[64] Marchetti P, Fovez Q, Germain N, Khamari R, Kluza J. Mitochondrial spare respiratory capacity: Mechanisms, regulation, and significance in non-transformed and cancer cells. The FASEB Journal. 2020;**34**(10):13106–13124

[65] Brand MD, Nicholls DG. Assessing mitochondrial dysfunction in cells. The Biochemical Journal. 2011;**435**(2):297–312

[66] Yadava N, Nicholls DG. Spare respiratory capacity rather than oxidative stress regulates glutamate excitotoxicity after partial respiratory inhibition of mitochondrial complex I with rotenone. The Journal of Neuroscience. 2007;**27**(27):7310–7317

[67] Hussain SNA, Sandri M, Gouspillou G. Editorial: Autophagy and Mitophagy in Skeletal Muscle Health and Disease. Frontiers in Physiology. 2021;**12**:703458

[68] Zhang XJ, Chen S, Huang KX, Le WD. Why should autophagic flux be assessed? Acta Pharmacologica Sinica. 2013;**34**(5):595–599

[69] Xia Q, Huang X, Huang J, et al. The role of autophagy in skeletal muscle diseases. Frontiers in Physiology. 2021;**12**:638983

[70] Guan Y, Drake JC, Yan Z. Exercise-induced mitophagy in skeletal muscle and heart. Exercise and Sport Sciences Reviews. 2019;**47**(3):151–156

[71] Zeng Z, Liang J, Wu L, Zhang H, Lv J, Chen N. Exercise-induced autophagy suppresses sarcopenia through Akt/mTOR and Akt/FoxO3a signal pathways and AMPK-mediated mitochondrial quality control. Frontiers in Physiology. 2020;**11**:583478

[72] Iorio R Regulation of Mitophagy. Encyclopedia. 2021. Available from: https://encyclopedia.pub/entry/18430 [Accessed: 2026-April-17]

[73] Yun HR, Jo YH, Kim J, et al. Palmitoyl Protein Thioesterase 1 is essential for Myogenic Autophagy of C2C12 skeletal myoblast. Frontiers in Physiology. 2020;**11**:569221

[74] Pivtoraiko VN, Stone SL, Roth KA, Shacka JJ. Oxidative stress and autophagy in the regulation of lysosome-dependent neuron death. Antioxidants & Redox Signaling. 2009;**11**(3):481–496

[75] Rovini A. Tubulin-VDAC Interaction: Molecular basis for mitochondrial dysfunction in chemotherapy-induced peripheral neuropathy. Frontiers in Physiology. 2019;**10**:671

[76] Chen CCW, Erlich AT, Crilly MJ, Hood DA. Parkin is required for exercise-induced mitophagy in muscle: Impact of aging. American Journal of Physiology-Endocrinology and Metabolism. 2018;**315**(3):E404–e415

[77] Vetter L, Cortassa S, O'Rourke B, et al. Diabetes increases the vulnerability of the cardiac mitochondrial network to criticality. Frontiers in Physiology. 2020;**11**:175

[78] Iorio R, Celenza G, Petricca S. Mitophagy: Molecular mechanisms, new concepts on parkin activation and the emerging role of AMPK/ULK1 Axis. Cells. 2021;**11**(1):30

[79] Seabright AP, Lai Y-C. Regulatory roles of PINK1-Parkin and AMPK in Ubiquitin-Dependent Skeletal Muscle Mitophagy. Frontiers in Physiology. 2020;**11**:608474

[80] Sanchez AMJ. Mitophagy flux in skeletal muscle during chronic contractile activity and ageing. The Journal of Physiology. 2018;**596**(16):3461–3462

[81] Lochner A, Wang H-H, Reiter RJ, Guo R, Hao Z. Editorial: Role of mitochondrial quality control in myocardial and microvascular physiology and pathophysiology. Frontiers in Physiology. 2021;**12**:745033

[82] Leipnitz G, Hatch GM, Mohsen A-W, Wanders RJA. Editorial: Mitochondrial disorders: Biochemical and molecular basis of disease. Frontiers in Genetics. 2021;**12**:769770

[83] Williams CF, George CH. Connect and conquer: Collectivized behavior of mitochondria and bacteria. Frontiers in Physiology. 2019;**10**:340

[84] Janssen JJE, Grefte S, Keijer J, de Boer VCJ. Mito-nuclear communication by mitochondrial metabolites and its regulation by B-Vitamins. Frontiers in Physiology. 2019;**10**:78

[85] Dakik P, Medkour Y, Mohammad K, Titorenko VI. Mechanisms through which some mitochondria-generated metabolites act as second messengers that are essential contributors to the aging process in eukaryotes across phyla. Frontiers in Physiology. 2019;**10**:461

[86] Milan G, Romanello V, Pescatore F, et al. Regulation of autophagy and the ubiquitin–proteasome system by the FoxO transcriptional network during muscle atrophy. Nature Communications 2015;**6**:6670

[87] Hajj-Boutros G, Karelis AD, Cefis M, et al. Potential mechanisms involved in regulating muscle protein turnover after acute exercise: A brief review. Frontiers in Physiology. 2023;**13**:1106425

[88] Thai PN, Seidlmayer LK, Miller C, et al. Mitochondrial quality control in aging and heart failure: Influence of ketone bodies and mitofusin-stabilizing peptides. Frontiers in Physiology. 2019;**10**:382

[89] Seidlmayer LK, Mages C, Berbner A, et al. Mitofusin 2 is essential for IP(3)-Mediated SR/Mitochondria metabolic feedback in ventricular myocytes. Frontiers in Physiology. 2019;**10**:733

[90] Youle RJ, van der Bliek AM. Mitochondrial fission, fusion, and stress. Science. 2012;**337**(6098):1062–1065

[91] Chatzinikita E, Maridaki M, Palikaras K, Koutsilieris M, Philippou A. The role of mitophagy in skeletal

muscle damage and regeneration. Cells. 2023;**12**(5):716

[92] Katti P, Kim Y, Sundaresan NR, Gouspillou G, Hinton A. Editorial: Muscle plasticity: Regulation of adaptive changes in muscles and mitochondrial dynamics. Frontiers in Physiology. 2023;**14**:1192759

[93] Yang J, Ran M, Li H, et al. New insight into neurological degeneration: Inflammatory cytokines and blood-brain barrier. Frontiers in Molecular Neuroscience. 2022;**15**:1013933

[94] Dantzer R, Konsman J-P, Bluthé R-M, Kelley KW. Neural and humoral pathways of communication from the immune system to the brain: Parallel or convergent? Autonomic Neuroscience. 2000;**85**(1):60–65

[95] Reyes R, Wu Y, Lai Q, et al. Early inflammatory response in rat brain after peripheral thermal injury. Neuroscience Letters 2006;**407**:11–15

[96] Herndon David N, Hart David W, Wolf Steven E, Chinkes David L, Wolfe Robert R. Reversal of catabolism by beta-blockade after severe burns. New England Journal of Medicine. 2001;**345** (17):1223–1229

[97] Norbury WB, Herndon DN, Branski LK, Chinkes DL, Jeschke MG. Urinary cortisol and catecholamine excretion after burn injury in children. The Journal of Clinical Endocrinology & Metabolism. 2008;**93**(4):1270–1275

[98] Tan JX, Finkel T. Mitochondria as intracellular signaling platforms in health and disease. The Journal of Cell Biology. 2020;**219**(5):e202002179

[99] Chen J, Kitagawa Y, Xie F, et al. Activated microglia mediate the motor neuron-, synaptic denervation- and muscle wasting-changes in burn injured mice. Journal of Cachexia, Sarcopenia and Muscle 2025;**16**:e13755

[100] Jena J, García-Peña LM, Pereira RO. The roles of FGF21 and GDF15 in mediating the mitochondrial integrated stress response. Frontiers in Endocrinology (Lausanne). 2023;**14**:1264530

[101] Kim J, Kim H-S, Chung JH. Molecular mechanisms of mitochondrial DNA release and activation of the cGAS-STING pathway. Experimental & Molecular Medicine. 2023;**55**(3):510–519

[102] Irazoki A, Gordaliza-Alaguero I, Frank E, et al. Disruption of mitochondrial dynamics triggers muscle inflammation through interorganellar contacts and mitochondrial DNA mislocation. Nature Communications 2023;**14**:108

[103] Nakazawa H, Ikeda K, Shinozaki S, et al. Coenzyme Q10 protects against burn-induced mitochondrial dysfunction and impaired insulin signaling in mouse skeletal muscle. FEBS Open Bio 2019;**9**:348–363

[104] Mao XJ, Li XS, Wang L, et al. Coenzyme Q10 mitigates high-fat-induced mitochondrial damage in spotted seabass (Lateolabrax maculatus) hepatocytes by promoting mitophagy. International Journal of Biological Macromolecules 2025;**331**:148436

[105] Zheng D, Cui C, Ye C, et al. Coenzyme Q10 prevents RANKL-induced osteoclastogenesis by promoting autophagy via inactivation of the PI3K/AKT/mTOR and MAPK pathways. Brazilian Journal of Medical and Biological Research. 2024;**57**:e13474

Section 3

Special Clinical Considerations

Chapter 5

Burn Management in Children and Newborns

Yücel Pekal and Ayşe Büşra Pekal

Abstract

Burn injuries in children and newborns remain a major global health problem and continue to cause significant morbidity, mortality, and long-term disability. The majority of pediatric burns occur in domestic environments, with scald injuries being the most common mechanism in toddlers and infants, while flame-related burns are more frequently observed in older children and adolescents. Neonates are uniquely vulnerable to burn injuries due to immature skin barrier function, limited thermoregulation, and reduced physiological reserves. Even brief exposure to moderate heat sources may result in deep tissue injury during the neonatal period. Physiological immaturity in newborns, including impaired vascular autoregulation and reduced cardiac output, limits effective heat dissipation and increases the risk of extensive tissue damage. In critically ill neonates, compromised perfusion and immature immune responses further exacerbate burn-related complications. These age-specific differences necessitate a tailored approach to assessment, resuscitation, wound management, and rehabilitation. This chapter provides a comprehensive and up-to-date review of burn management in children and newborns, focusing on epidemiology, pathophysiology, classification, acute management, surgical intervention, nutritional support, rehabilitation, and prevention strategies. Emphasis is placed on age-specific clinical considerations and evidence-based practices aimed at improving survival and long-term functional outcomes.

Keywords: pediatric burns, neonatal burns, burn management, fluid resuscitation, wound care, pain management, rehabilitation, burn prevention

1. Introduction

Burn injuries represent one of the most common and devastating forms of accidental trauma in childhood. Despite substantial improvements in prevention, emergency care, and burn center management, pediatric burn injuries remain a significant cause of morbidity and long-term disability worldwide. Children who survive severe burns often experience prolonged hospitalization, repeated surgical procedures, growth disturbances, functional limitations, and psychological sequelae that may persist into adulthood [1].

Children are not simply small adults. Their anatomical, physiological, and developmental characteristics profoundly influence both the severity of burn injuries

IntechOpen

and the response to treatment. A higher body surface area-to-weight ratio predisposes children to greater fluid loss and heat dissipation, while limited physiological reserves increase their vulnerability to shock and organ dysfunction. Behavioral factors, such as curiosity and limited hazard awareness, further contribute to the risk of burns [2].

Newborns represent the most fragile subgroup within the pediatric population. The immaturity of the skin barrier, underdeveloped thermoregulation, immature renal and immune function, and dependence on caregivers for protection significantly increase the risk of severe injury. Burn management in neonates requires meticulous attention to detail and should ideally be conducted in specialized neonatal or pediatric intensive care units [3].

2. Epidemiology

Burn injuries affect millions of children globally each year. According to recent data from the World Health Organization, pediatric burns remain a leading cause of injury-related morbidity, particularly in low- and middle-income countries where access to preventive measures and specialized burn care is limited [1]. In high-income countries, more than 100,000 children require hospital-based care annually for burn injuries, although mortality rates have declined over recent decades.

Age is a major determinant of burn etiology. In infants and toddlers younger than three years, scald injuries account for approximately 60–70% of burns. These injuries commonly occur in domestic environments, particularly kitchens and bathrooms, and are frequently associated with hot liquids, bathing accidents, or overturned containers. Flame burns become more prevalent in school-aged children and adolescents, often related to house fires, outdoor activities, or the unsafe use of flammable materials.

Neonatal burns are rare but often severe when they occur. Common causes include contact with heating devices, accidental exposure to hot surfaces, extravasation injuries, and iatrogenic burns related to medical equipment. Socioeconomic status, housing conditions, parental supervision, and caregiver education significantly influence burn risk, highlighting the importance of targeted prevention strategies.

3. Pathophysiology of burn injury

Burn injury initiates a complex cascade of local and systemic physiological responses. Thermal damage to the skin and underlying tissues results in coagulative necrosis, increased capillary permeability, and the release of inflammatory mediators. These changes lead to plasma leakage into the interstitial space, causing edema and intravascular volume depletion.

Extensive burns involving more than 20% of the total body surface area (TBSA) may trigger systemic inflammatory response syndrome (SIRS). This systemic response is characterized by tachycardia, an increased metabolic rate, insulin resistance, and immune dysregulation. Prolonged hypermetabolism results in muscle protein catabolism, impaired wound healing, and increased susceptibility to infection [4].

Children experience a more pronounced hypermetabolic response compared to adults. Limited energy reserves, combined with increased nutritional requirements for growth, exacerbate the negative impact of prolonged inflammation and catabolism.

3.1 Pathophysiological differences in newborns

Neonatal skin differs structurally and functionally from that of older children and adults. The stratum corneum is thinner and contains less lipid, resulting in reduced barrier function and increased transepidermal water loss. These characteristics allow thermal energy to penetrate more deeply, increasing the likelihood of full-thickness injury.

Thermoregulatory mechanisms in neonates are immature. Autonomic nervous system immaturity impairs vasoconstriction and vasodilation responses, limiting the ability to conserve or dissipate heat effectively. As a result, neonates are at high risk of hypothermia during both the initial injury and subsequent treatment.

Renal immaturity restricts the ability to concentrate urine and regulate electrolytes, complicating fluid resuscitation. In addition, neonatal immune responses are underdeveloped, increasing susceptibility to infection and sepsis. These factors necessitate individualized treatment strategies and continuous monitoring.

4. Classification of burns

Burn injuries are classified according to depth, extent, and etiology. Accurate classification is essential for guiding management decisions and predicting outcomes.

4.1 Classification by depth

Superficial burns: Involve only the epidermis and typically heal without scarring.

Partial-thickness burns: Extend into the dermis and may be superficial or deep, with variable healing potential.

Full-thickness burns: Involve the entire dermis and require surgical intervention.

Deep burns: Extend into fascia, muscle, or bone, and are associated with high morbidity.

4.2 Classification by extent

Burn size is expressed as a percentage of TBSA. In pediatric patients, the Lund–Browder chart is preferred because it accounts for age-related differences in body proportions.

4.3 Classification by etiology

Burns may result from thermal, electrical, chemical, radiation, or friction mechanisms, each presenting distinct clinical challenges.

5. Initial assessment and stabilization

Initial management follows the ABCDE trauma approach. Early airway assessment is critical, particularly in suspected inhalation injury. Breathing and oxygenation should be evaluated promptly, with supplemental oxygen administered as needed. Circulatory status must be assessed rapidly, intravenous access established, and fluid resuscitation initiated without delay.

Preventing hypothermia during exposure and examination is especially important in infants and neonates.

6. Fluid resuscitation

Adequate fluid resuscitation is a cornerstone of burn management. The Parkland formula remains the most widely used method for estimating initial fluid requirements:

4 mL × body weight (kg) × %TBSA burned

Half of the calculated volume is administered within the first 8 hours after injury, with the remaining half given over the subsequent 16 hours [2, 5].

6.1 Pediatric considerations

Children require the addition of maintenance fluids to resuscitation volumes. Glucose-containing solutions are essential in infants to prevent hypoglycemia. Target urine output is 0.5–1 mL/kg/hour in older children and 1–2 mL/kg/hour in neonates.

6.2 Avoiding over-resuscitation

Excessive fluid administration, often referred to as "fluid creep," may result in pulmonary edema, abdominal compartment syndrome, and worsening tissue edema. Close monitoring of urine output, lactate levels, and hemodynamic parameters is essential.

7. Pain management

Pain control is fundamental to burn care. Uncontrolled pain increases stress responses, delays healing, and negatively affects psychological outcomes. A multimodal approach is recommended, combining pharmacological and non-pharmacological strategies.

Paracetamol, opioids, and ketamine are commonly used agents. In neonates, oral sucrose, minimal handling, and environmental control provide additional comfort.

8. Wound care

Optimal wound care promotes healing and prevents infection. Initial management includes gentle cleansing, removal of debris, and early debridement of nonviable tissue. Topical antimicrobial agents and modern dressings should be selected based on burn depth and exudate.

Silver-containing products should be used cautiously in neonates due to the risk of systemic absorption [6].

9. Surgical management

Surgical intervention is indicated for deep and extensive burns. Early excision and split-thickness skin grafting reduce the risk of infection and shorten hospitalization. Escharotomy is required in circumferential burns with vascular compromise, and fasciotomy may be necessary in cases of compartment syndrome [7].

10. Special considerations in newborns

Neonatal burn management requires continuous thermal support, strict fluid and electrolyte monitoring, weight-based drug dosing, and frequent reassessment. Care should be provided in specialized neonatal intensive care units whenever possible.

11. Nutritional support

Early enteral feeding within 6–12 hours post-injury is recommended. High-protein nutrition supports wound healing and counteracts hypermetabolism. In neonates, breast milk is preferred, with fortification as needed [8].

12. Complications

Burn-related complications include sepsis, acute respiratory distress syndrome, acute kidney injury, hypertrophic scarring, and contractures. Early recognition and aggressive management improve outcomes.

13. Rehabilitation and long-term care

Rehabilitation should begin early and include physical therapy, range-of-motion exercises, pressure garments, silicone therapy, and psychological support. Long-term follow-up is essential to address functional and psychosocial outcomes.

14. Prevention

Prevention remains the most effective strategy to reduce the pediatric burn burden. Home safety education, hot water temperature regulation, smoke detector installation, and neonatal unit safety protocols are critical components.

15. Conclusions

Burn management in children and newborns requires a prompt, multidisciplinary, and age-specific approach. Understanding developmental differences in physiology and response to injury is essential for optimizing care. Early stabilization, appropriate resuscitation, meticulous wound management, nutritional support, and rehabilitation significantly improve survival and long-term quality of life.

Acknowledgments

The authors acknowledge the use of ChatGPT (OpenAI) for language editing and stylistic refinement of the chapter. The scientific content, clinical interpretations, and final responsibility for the manuscript remain entirely with the authors.

Conflict of Interest

The authors declare no conflict of interest.

Author details

Yücel Pekal[1*] and Ayşe Büşra Pekal[2]

1 Department of Neonatology, Denizli State Hospital, Denizli, Türkiye

2 Department of Child Neurology, Pamukkale University Faculty of Medicine Hospital, Denizli, Türkiye

*Address all correspondence to: kardiyak5410@gmail.com

References

[1] World Health Organization. Global Burn Registry Report. Geneva: WHO; 2023. Available from: https://www.who.int/teams/social-determinants-of-health/safety-and-mobility/burns/global-burn-registry [Accessed: 2026-April-24]

[2] Greenhalgh DG. Management of burns. New England Journal of Medicine. 2019;**380**:2349–2359. DOI: 10.1056/NEJMra1807442

[3] Sheridan RL. Burns in Children. Journal of Burn Care & Research. 2017;**38**(3):e618–e624. DOI: 10.1097/BCR.0000000000000536

[4] Jeschke MG, van Baar ME, Choudhry MA, et al. Burn injury. Nature Reviews Disease Primers. 2020;**6**:11

[5] Kraft Casey T, Agarwal S, Ranganathan K, Wong VW, Loder S, Li J, Delano MJ, Levi B. Trauma-induced heterotopic bone formation and the role of the immune system: A review. Journal of Trauma and Acute Care Surgery. 2016;**80**(1):156–165. DOI: 10.1097/TA.0000000000000883

[6] Shah AR, Liao LF. Pediatric Burn Care: Unique Considerations in Management. Clinics in Plastic Surgery. 2017;**44**(3):603–610. DOI: 10.1016/j.cps.2017.02.017

[7] Pham TN, Cancio LC, Gibran NS. American Burn Association Practice Guidelines Burn Shock Resuscitation. Journal of Burn Care & Research. 2008;**29**(1):257–266. DOI: 10.1097/BCR.0b013e31815f3876

[8] Williams FN, Branski LK, Jeschke MG, Herndon DN. What, how, and how much should patients with burns be fed?. Surgical Clinics of North America. 2011;**91**(3):609–29. DOI: 10.1016/j.suc.2011.03.002

Chapter 6

Electrical Burn

Emily Vanderpool, Maysa Shemmiyeva and Desmond Khor

Abstract

Electrical injuries occupy a unique intersection between burn, trauma, and critical care medicine, where varied mechanisms, unpredictable clinical trajectories, and a high risk of multisystem complications influence treatment decisions. Unlike conventional thermal burns, the severity of injury is often poorly reflected by external findings, as electrical current may produce extensive multi system internal tissue damage. Variability in voltage, current type, exposure duration, and tissue resistance contributes to a wide spectrum of clinical presentations, ranging from minor cutaneous injury to life-threatening organ dysfunction. This chapter synthesizes current evidence on the pathophysiology, clinical manifestations, and management of electrical burn injuries, with an emphasis on critical care considerations. Foundational principles of electrical injury, including mechanisms of tissue damage and patterns of associated injury, are discussed to provide context for risk stratification and early recognition. Key components of intensive care unit management are examined, including cardiac monitoring, fluid resuscitation strategies tailored to rhabdomyolysis, neurologic surveillance, and respiratory support. Surgical management principles such as early recognition of compartment syndrome, serial wound assessment, and timely operative intervention are also reviewed. In addition, common cardiovascular, metabolic, infectious, and long-term complications are outlined to highlight the need for multidisciplinary care and longitudinal follow-up. By integrating mechanistic understanding with contemporary critical care and surgical practices, this chapter provides a structured framework for clinicians managing patients with electrical injuries. Emphasis is placed on recognizing occult injury, anticipating delayed complications, and applying coordinated multidisciplinary strategies to improve outcomes in this complex patient population.

Keywords: electrical injury, burn injury, wounds, lightning injury, electrical burn

1. Introduction

Electrical injuries represent a distinct form of trauma characterized by heterogeneous mechanisms and highly variable clinical trajectories. Although they account for a smaller proportion of overall burn admissions than thermal burns, these injuries often carry disproportionate morbidity due to their potential for hidden tissue damage, multisystem involvement, and delayed complications. Occupational exposures remain a major contributor in industrialized settings, particularly among working-age adults, while household accidents and high-risk environmental encounters contribute to injuries across other age groups. Limitations in reporting and inconsistent epidemiological data suggest that the true burden of electrical trauma is likely underrecognized.

Unlike conventional thermal burns, electrical injuries blur traditional boundaries between burn surgery, trauma care, and critical care medicine. Patients may present with minimal external findings yet develop significant neurologic, cardiovascular, or musculoskeletal sequelae, creating diagnostic and management challenges across the continuum of care. The variability in presentation has historically led to inconsistent classification and treatment strategies; therefore, a framework that integrates mechanistic understanding with modern multidisciplinary management is needed.

The initial sections herein outline the foundational principles that shape injury patterns and clinical manifestations, providing context for risk recognition and early evaluation. Subsequent sections focus on intensive care management, surgical decision-making, and the prevention of acute and delayed complications, with dedicated consideration of lightning injury as a distinct clinical entity. By separating mechanistic context from management strategy, this chapter aims to provide a practical and clinically oriented synthesis for providers caring for patients with electrical burn injuries.

2. Incidence, prevalence, and risk factors

Electrical injuries result in complex pathologies that demand specialized clinical expertise. Between 2021 and 2022, the U.S. Bureau of Labor Statistics reported 3,260 occupational electrical injuries necessitating time away from work, with 36% of these cases involving men aged 25–34 (**Figure 1**, **Table 1**) [1]. Notably, 890 of these incidents resulted in more than 31 days of lost productivity.

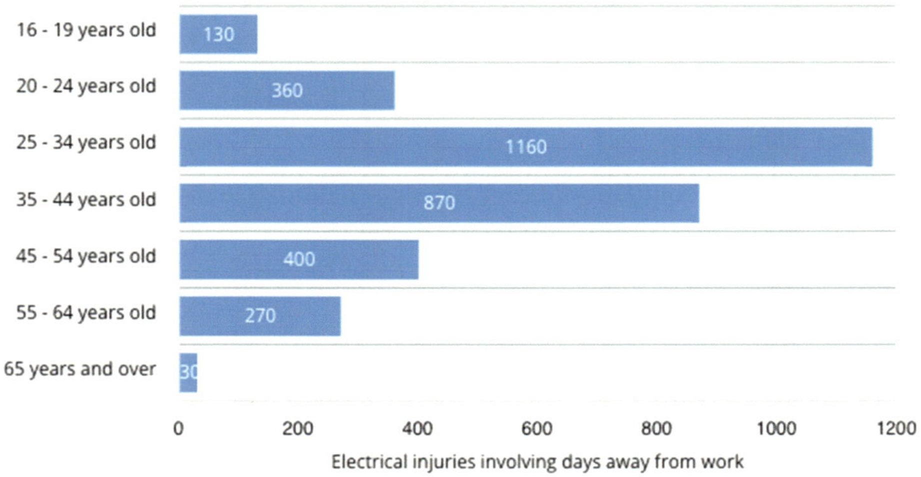

Figure 1.
Non-fatal electrical injuries by age of worker, Bureau of Labor Statistics, 2021–2022 [1].

Current (mA)	Response
0.2–2	"Electrical" sensation
1–2+	Painful shock
3–5	Let-go threshold for children
6–10	Minimum let-go threshold for adults
22	99% of adults cannot let go.
10–20	Tetany (contact area)
20–50	Tetany (respiratory muscles)
50–100	Ventricular fibrillation

Table 1.
Physical effects at selected currents [10].

However, these figures significantly underestimate the true global burden. The incidence of electrical injury follows a distinct trimodal distribution across different age groups and environments. The first peak occurs in young children, who experience high levels of accidental household exposures, typically involving low-voltage outlets or appliances. The second peak involves adolescent males, whose injuries are often the result of risk-seeking behaviors such as train surfing or climbing high-voltage structures. Finally, the third peak is seen in adult males between the ages of 20 and 45, where the burden of injury is driven predominantly by occupational exposures in industrial or construction settings. Many lower-voltage household exposures never reach medical attention, further obscuring the data. While literature frequently cites that electrical injuries comprise 5% of all burn admissions [2–6], reference tracing suggests this figure may be outdated, originating from an analysis of 1991–1993 ABA registry data [7]. Consequently, the current and true impact of electrical injuries remains clinically underappreciated.

3. Pathophysiology

The severity of an electrical injury is fundamentally governed by the physics of the exposure, specifically Ohm's Law, which states that current (I) travels proportionally to voltage (V) and inversely to tissue resistance (R) [Eq. (1)]. Joule's law further explains that the power (P), or heat generation from this exposure, is multiplicative – a product of exponentiated current and resistance [Eq. (2)]. Consequently, tissues with higher resistance may sustain greater thermal injury regardless of how they appear superficially.

$$\text{Ohm's Law: Current (I)} = \text{Voltage (V)/Resistance (R)} \tag{1}$$

$$\text{Joule's Law: Power (J [Joules])} = \text{Current}^2(\text{I}^2)\ \text{x Resistance (R)} \tag{2}$$

The specific characteristics of the current source add a layer of nuance to these injuries. In North America, Alternating Current (AC) cyclically changes the direction of electron flow at 60 Hz and is commonly found in household wiring, while Direct Current (DC) maintains a unidirectional flow and is found in batteries, cars, and high-voltage sources like subway third rails [6, 8]. These types differ in their physical impact: AC exposure is connected to the "no let-go" effect, where tetanic muscular contraction prevents the victim from releasing the contact point, thereby increasing exposure duration. Conversely, DC exposure often causes a "jump back" effect, where a singular strong contraction throws the victim away from the source. While this may decrease exposure time, it increases the prevalence of blunt force traumas, such as fractures [8, 9].

As the current moves through the body, the internal damage is dictated by the resistance of specific tissues. Nerve tissue typically has the least resistance and may be damaged even at low voltages without cutaneous manifestations. Blood and vascular tissue also have low resistance, followed by muscle, while bone and fat possess the highest resistance. Because energy is lost to high-resistance tissue in the form of heat, these areas often suffer coagulation necrosis [10]. Furthermore, the spreading and distortion of current, known as volume conduction, lead to more severe injuries in body parts with smaller cross-sectional areas, such as the ankles and wrists [9, 11].

At the cellular level, the flow of current causes electroporation of cell membranes. This process forms aqueous pores, making it impossible for the membrane to maintain the critical ionic difference between the cytoplasm and extracellular space. The resulting influx of ions, such as calcium, triggers apoptosis, with the elongated structure of muscle and nerve cells proving most vulnerable [9, 12]. Additionally, electrical exposure can alter the polarity of amino acids and change the functionality of voltage-gated channel proteins [9, 13].

Clinically, these exposures are regularly classified into low-voltage (<1000 V) and high-voltage (< 1000 V) and high voltage (>>1000 V) categories. The overall severity is contingent on the intensity, type, voltage, contact resistance, duration, and pathway of the current within the body [14]. High-voltage exposure is more often associated with acute sequelae, though acute paralysis and neurological symptoms at presentation are often associated with a better recovery than cases involving a delayed presentation [15]. These mechanisms explain the high incidence of cardiac and neurologic dysfunction described in later clinical sections.

In contrast to current exposure, electrical arcing is a dangerous discharge of current in which electricity jumps a gap and ionizes the air into plasma. Arcing creates intense heat (often over 10,000 °F), bright light, and sparks that can lead to both fire and/or electrical shock. Faulty wiring, loose connection points, or overloaded circuits are common causes of electrical arcs. Arcing can also be induced by a grounded object (i.e., a person) simply approaching a cable carrying high voltage [16]. Arc injuries are commonly associated with flash and flame burns, blunt force traumas induced by a similar "jump back" effect to that seen in DC current exposures, and acoustic trauma, such as ruptured eardrums (**Table 2**).

4. Clinical presentation

Patients with electrical injuries present unique diagnostic and therapeutic challenges, as their clinical manifestations range from minor cutaneous burns to catastrophic internal organ damage. These injuries often involve a complex interplay of thermal, electrophysiological, traumatic, and metabolic derangements that can affect every organ system. Early recognition is frequently complicated by the fact

Low-voltage shock effects (<600 Volts)	**High-voltage shock effects (600 + Volts)**
Superficial burns	Deep and occult burns
No late arrhythmia	Case reports of late arrhythmia
Usually alternating current	Either alternating current or direct current.
Rhabdomyolysis uncommon	Rhabdomyolysis common
Secondary trauma less common	Secondary trauma from falls and tetanic muscle contractions
Contact is prolonged (unable to let go)	Contact can be brief (thrown from the voltage source)
Cardiac arrest from ventricular fibrillation	Cardiac arrest from ventricular fibrillation; direct damage to the myocardium, causing asystole; and coronary artery thrombosis

Table 2.
Effects of Low Voltage Versus High Voltage Electrical Shock [10].

that patients may present with symptoms resembling those of standard cardiac, trauma, or burn victims, often in the absence of a clear clinical history [10].

The local pathology of an electrical current injury typically manifests as an electrochemical burn at the contact site, characterized by a center of charred tissue. Crucially, the external severity of these burns does not always correlate with the magnitude of the voltage because exposure duration acts as a multiplier of total tissue damage. This is particularly evident in high-voltage exposures, where patients may lack significant superficial burns despite harboring extensive deep-tissue destruction beneath relatively uninjured skin [10].

Beyond visible wounds, the multi-system impact of the current can trigger cardiac arrhythmias, seizures, paresthesia, and various sensory or motor deficits. Because the underlying cellular damage is often progressive, symptoms may be delayed in onset, necessitating prolonged clinical observation and repeated evaluation.

5. Associated injuries

Electrical injuries produce a broad spectrum of associated systemic complications that reflect the preferential flow of current through neural and vascular tissues. Neurologic involvement is common, particularly following high-voltage exposure, with loss of consciousness representing the most frequent acute manifestation [5]. Direct neural injury may affect both central and peripheral pathways, often involving proprioceptive fibers, and patients may develop seizures, persistent sensory deficits, neuropathic pain, or delayed neuropsychological changes, including impairments in memory, attention, and behavior [2, 15].

Cardiovascular complications arise when electrical current traverses the thorax or major vascular structures [9, 17]. The myocardium is highly susceptible to electrical disruption, predisposing patients to arrhythmias, conduction abnormalities, or sudden cardiac arrest [18]. These effects may occur even in low-voltage exposures and may not correlate with the severity of cutaneous injury [19].

Deep tissue injury frequently evolves over time due to progressive vascular compromise and ongoing muscle necrosis along the current pathway. This process may culminate in compartment syndrome or extensive rhabdomyolysis, particularly in muscle groups adjacent to bone where resistance is greatest. Associated metabolic disturbances and renal dysfunction may develop as secondary consequences of myonecrosis [10, 20].

Secondary traumatic injuries are also common. Tetanic muscle contraction or blast forces generated by electrical exposure may result in fractures, joint dislocations, or spinal injury, while falls contribute additional blunt trauma [21]. Long-term sequelae may include sensorineural hearing loss, vertigo, and ocular complications such as cataract formation, often ipsilateral to the entry site [15, 22]. Because many of these manifestations evolve gradually, their relationship to the initial electrical exposure may be overlooked without careful clinical correlation [15].

While the early sections describe the biological and clinical manifestations of electrical injury, the following sections focus on ICU-level management strategies driven by the unique risks of occult tissue necrosis and delayed systemic complications.

6. Intensive care unit management of electrical burn patients

Electrical burn injuries constitute a distinct and highly complex subset of burn trauma, in which the extent of internal injury is frequently disproportionate to the external cutaneous findings. Early series by Purdue and Hunt demonstrated that significant deep tissue necrosis, cardiac arrhythmias, renal failure, and neurologic injury may occur despite limited skin involvement [23]. Subsequent reviews and practice guidelines have reinforced the need for early intensive care unit (ICU) admission for patients with moderate to severe electrical injuries due to the high incidence of multisystem complications [17, 24, 25]. Indications for ICU admission in electrical burn patients are summarized in **Table 3**.

6.1 Initial stabilization and monitoring

Initial management must follow Advanced Trauma Life Support (ATLS) principles, with immediate attention to airway protection, cervical spine

Indication	Rationale
High-voltage exposure (>1000 V)	Increased risk of deep tissue necrosis, arrhythmias.
Loss of consciousness or cardiac arrest	Risk of delayed arrhythmias and neurologic injury
Abnormal ECG or dysrhythmia	Possible myocardial injury requiring monitoring
Evidence of rhabdomyolysis (elevated CK, myoglobinuria).	Increased risk of acute kidney injury
Neurologic deficits	Potential central or peripheral nerve injury
Extensive soft tissue injury or compartment syndrome	Need for serial examinations and possible surgical intervention
Lightning strike	Risk of cardiopulmonary arrest and delayed neurologic sequelae

Table 3.
ICU admission indications for electrical burn injuries.

immobilization when indicated, and circulatory stabilization. High-voltage exposure, loss of consciousness, or associated blunt trauma mandates a full trauma evaluation, as emphasized in the American Burn Association (ABA) and Joint Trauma System (JTS) guidelines [17, 26].

Continuous cardiac monitoring is mandatory in all patients with significant electrical exposure. AC is particularly arrhythmogenic and may induce both immediate and delayed dysrhythmias, including ventricular fibrillation, atrial fibrillation, and conduction disturbances [12, 27]. Koumbourlis and the ABA guidelines recommend continuous electrocardiographic (ECG) monitoring for a minimum of 24 hours, which should be extended in patients with loss of consciousness, abnormal initial ECG, or high-voltage exposure [17, 25].

Invasive arterial blood pressure monitoring should be considered in patients with hemodynamic instability, major associated trauma, or extensive tissue injury, consistent with modern burn ICU protocols [26, 28].

6.2 Fluid resuscitation and renal protection

Deep muscle necrosis with myoglobin release is a defining pathophysiologic feature of electrical burns. Lee et al. demonstrated that electrical current produces direct myocyte membrane injury, predisposing individuals to extensive rhabdomyolysis even in the absence of large surface burns [12]. Rhabdomyolysis is a major contributor to acute kidney injury (AKI), which remains a leading cause of morbidity in this population [24, 29].

Early and aggressive crystalloid resuscitation is, therefore, essential. Standard burn formulas frequently underestimate fluid needs in high-voltage injuries, and several authors advocate for higher urine output (UOP) targets than those used in thermal burns [24, 29, 30].

Recommended targets include:

- Urine output ≥ 1–1.5 mL/kg/hr in all electrical burn patients [17, 24]

- Urine output ≥ 2 mL/kg/hr in patients with established rhabdomyolysis or myoglobinuria [29, 30]

Serial monitoring of creatine kinase (CK), serum myoglobin, electrolytes, arterial blood gases, and urine characteristics is essential to guide resuscitation and detect evolving renal dysfunction [17, 25, 30]. Urine alkalinization and osmotic diuresis with mannitol have been proposed; however, evidence remains mixed, and these strategies should be applied selectively [17, 30].

6.3 Neurologic and respiratory care

Neurologic injury following electrical exposure may be immediate or delayed and may involve the central or peripheral nervous system. Arnoldo and Purdue reported delayed neurologic deterioration occurring weeks to months after injury, emphasizing the need for longitudinal surveillance [24]. As previously mentioned, manifestations include altered mental status, seizures, peripheral neuropathy, spinal cord injury, and progressive myelopathy [12, 25].

Frequent neurologic examinations are mandatory in the ICU. Early neuroimaging is indicated in patients with focal deficits, altered consciousness, or suspected spinal involvement, consistent with ABA and trauma guidelines [17]. Respiratory failure may result from associated trauma, aspiration, neurogenic mechanisms, or massive fluid shifts. Early mechanical ventilation should be instituted when indicated, following standard critical care principles [26].

7. Medical and surgical management and complications

7.1 Wound evaluation and surgical management

Electrical burns characteristically produce small points of contact wounds with extensive underlying tissue destruction along the current pathway. Early surgical series emphasized that reliance on skin findings alone leads to an underestimation of injury severity [23, 24]. Serial wound assessments and a low threshold for serial operative exploration/debridement are, therefore, critical.

Indications for early operative intervention include:

- Suspected compartment syndrome
- Progressive limb ischemia
- Deep muscle necrosis
- Evidence of infection

Fasciotomy is recommended when compartment syndrome is suspected, as delayed decompression is associated with irreversible neuromuscular injury [17, 24]. Aggressive debridement of devitalized muscle and soft tissue reduces the risk of infection and systemic toxicity [23, 24]. Reconstruction typically requires delayed closure, split-thickness skin grafting, or flap coverage, depending on the extent and depth of injury. Amputation may be required in cases of irreversible myonecrosis, major vascular injury, or uncontrolled infection – a finding consistently reported in long-term cohort studies [23, 24, 31].

The images in **Figure 2** demonstrate the profound deep tissue destruction that may occur in electrical burn injuries. Despite variable cutaneous involvement, extensive muscle necrosis, compartment injury, and progressive devitalization are evident upon surgical exploration. These photographs underscore the frequently deceptive external appearance of electrical trauma and the necessity for vigilant clinical and operative evaluation.

7.2 Cardiovascular and vascular complications

Direct myocardial injury, coronary spasm, and delayed arrhythmias have been described following both low- and high-voltage exposure [12, 25, 27]. Continuous telemetry remains the cornerstone of early detection [17, 25].

Electrical current may also cause vascular thrombosis and delayed ischemia. Vascular imaging is indicated in patients with pulse deficits, asymmetric perfusion, or progressive tissue ischemia [17, 24]. Late vascular complications, including

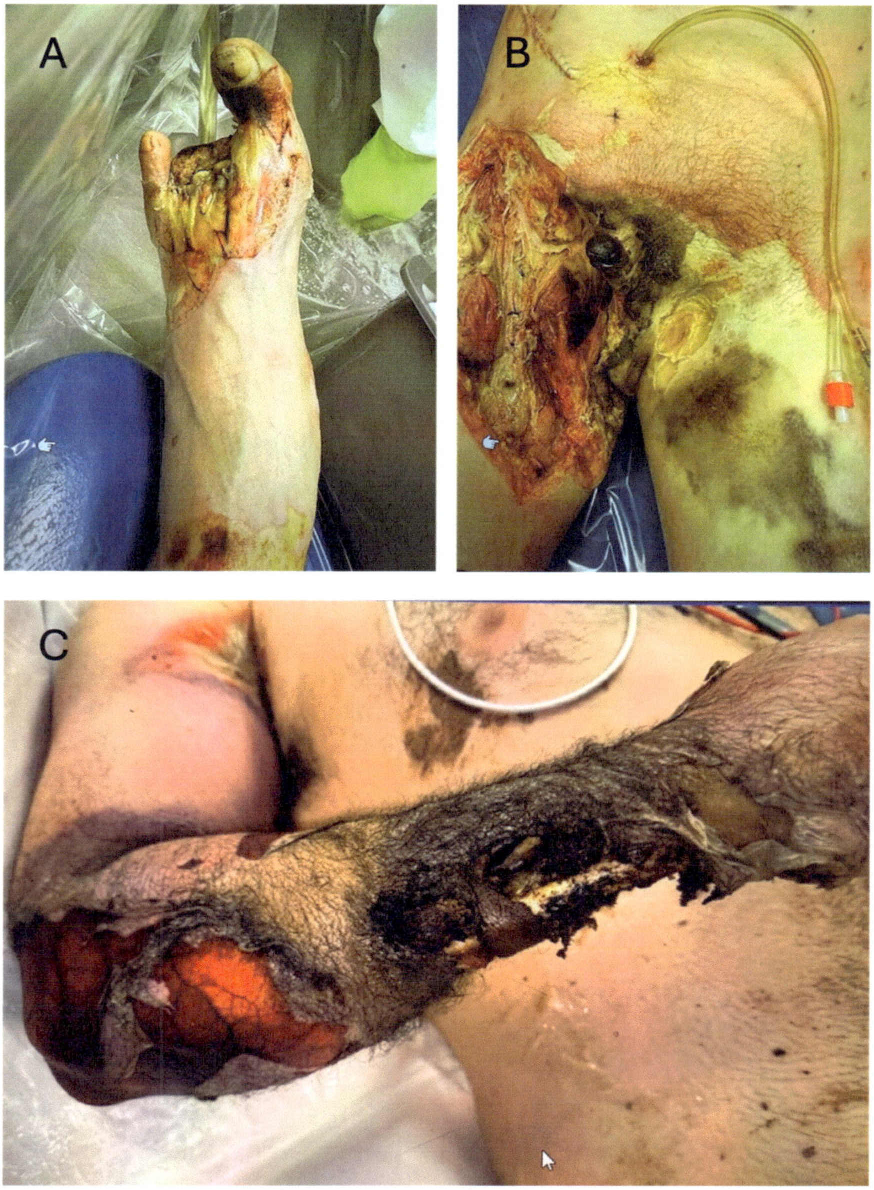

Figure 2.
Representative Cases of Electrical Burn Injury.

pseudoaneurysm formation, have been described and warrant surveillance in selected patients [17, 24].

7.3 Infectious and metabolic complications

Electrical burn patients are at an increased risk for wound infection, sepsis, electrolyte derangements, and metabolic acidosis [17, 24]. Common metabolic

System	Complication
Cardiovascular	Ventricular arrhythmias, conduction abnormalities, myocardial necrosis
Renal	Rhabdomyolysis, acute kidney injury
Neurologic	Peripheral neuropathy, spinal cord injury, seizures, delayed paralysis
Musculoskeletal	Compartment syndrome, myonecrosis, fractures
Vascular	Thrombosis, delayed ischemia, pseudoaneurysm
Ocular	Cataract formation
Psychiatric	Post-traumatic stress disorder (PTSD), depression, cognitive impairment

Table 4.
Common Complications of Electrical Injury.

abnormalities include hyperkalemia, hypocalcemia, and lactic acidosis secondary to muscle necrosis and shock [25, 29]. Early enteral nutrition, strict glycemic control, and structured infection surveillance are essential components of burn care, consistent with modern burn management guidelines [17, 26].

7.4 Long-term and delayed complications

Survivors of electrical injury may experience a range of long-term complications, including chronic pain syndromes; neuropsychiatric sequelae characterized by somatic, cognitive, and emotional impairments, as well as newly diagnosed psychiatric disorders; progressive neurologic deficits such as peripheral neuropathy, paresthesia, partial or complete paralysis; and cataract formation, particularly following high-voltage or lightning exposure, as summarized in **Table 4** [5, 24, 25, 32]. Although neurologic and neuropsychological recovery is possible, optimal functional outcomes require multidisciplinary follow-up involving burn surgery, neurology, psychiatry, ophthalmology, and rehabilitation medicine [17, 24].

Electrical injuries can also interfere with returning to gainful employment. A previous study reported that only 30%–60% of patients successfully return to work, with the majority requiring duty or schedule modifications due to newly diagnosed musculoskeletal or neuropsychiatric symptoms [5].

8. Special considerations: Lightning injury

8.1 Pathophysiology

Lightning injuries represent a unique form of electrical trauma, characterized by extremely high voltage, short duration, and predominantly superficial current flow over the body surface (the flashover phenomenon) (**Table 5**). Cooper et al. and subsequent Wilderness Medical Society (WMS) guidelines demonstrated that deep tissue necrosis is uncommon, while cardiopulmonary and neurologic effects predominate [32, 33].

The primary cause of death is cardiorespiratory arrest. Lichtenberg figures, like those in **Figure 3**, are pathognomonic but transient and do not represent true burns [32,33].

Feature	Electrical injury	Lightning injury
Voltage	Variable (often lower)	Extremely high
Duration	Prolonged contact	Milliseconds
Tissue Damage	Deep muscle and organ injury	Predominately superficial (flashover)
Mortality	Related to the extent of injury	Related to initial arrest
Skin Findings	Point of contact wounds	Lichtenburg figures
Surgical Need	Common	Rare

Table 5.
Key Differences: Electrical vs. Lightning Injury.

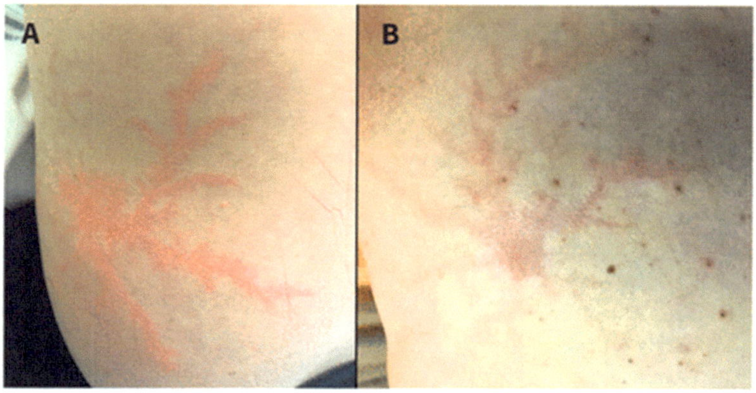

Figure 3.
Lichtenberg figures from lightning injury [37].

8.2 Clinical presentation

Common manifestations include immediate loss of consciousness, cardiac arrhythmias or asystole, respiratory arrest, tympanic membrane rupture, and focal or diffuse neurologic deficits [32, 34, 35].

8.3 Management principles

Management priorities differ from industrial electrical injuries. Immediate cardiopulmonary resuscitation is paramount. Both the WMS guidelines and AHA “Special Circumstances” statements emphasize that prolonged resuscitation may be successful and advocate reverse triage, prioritizing apneic and pulseless patients first [33, 36]

Survivors require monitoring for delayed neurologic deterioration. Neurologic complications include seizures, paresthesia, and paralysis, which can be transient in nature. Altered mental status or low Glasgow Coma Scale (GCS) should raise suspicion for underlying traumatic brain injury and should prompt appropriate evaluation and management [9].

Cutaneous burns are typically superficial and managed conservatively [32, 34, 35].

8.4 Prognosis

Despite the dramatic presentation, patients who survive the initial arrest may have favorable long-term outcomes with appropriate supportive care, although delayed neurologic and cognitive sequelae are well-documented [32, 34, 35].

9. Conclusion

Electrical injuries remain among the most complex and unpredictable forms of burn trauma, distinguished by mechanisms that extend beyond cutaneous damage to involve deep tissue, neurologic, cardiovascular, and metabolic systems. The clinical course is often defined by occult injury progression and delayed complications, underscoring the limitations of traditional burn assessment strategies that rely primarily on surface findings. Recognition of the unique pathophysiology of electrical exposure is, therefore, essential for early risk stratification and appropriate escalation of care.

Management requires a multidisciplinary approach that integrates trauma principles, burn surgery, and critical care medicine. Continuous cardiac monitoring, vigilant neurological assessment, and resuscitation strategies tailored to rhabdomyolysis and evolving tissue injury are central components of early management, while timely surgical intervention remains critical in preventing irreversible neuromuscular damage. Long-term follow-up is equally important, as survivors frequently experience persistent neurological, sensory, and functional sequelae that may emerge well after the acute phase of injury.

Despite advances in critical care and surgical techniques, significant gaps remain in the contemporary understanding of electrical injury epidemiology, optimal resuscitation targets, and predictors of delayed complications. Much of the existing literature is derived from retrospective series, reflecting the need for prospective, multicenter investigations and standardized reporting frameworks. Future work should focus on refining risk stratification, improving early diagnostic tools for deep tissue injury, and developing evidence-based protocols tailored specifically to electrical trauma. By aligning mechanistic insight with structured critical care and surgical management, clinicians can better anticipate complications and improve outcomes for patients affected by this uniquely challenging form of injury.

Acknowledgments

The authors would like to thank the University Medical Center (UMC) Foundation in Lubbock, Texas, for financially supporting this work.

The authors also acknowledge the use of ChatGPT for language editing in the chapter.

Conflict of Interest

The authors declare no conflict of interest.

Author details

Emily Vanderpool, Maysa Shemmiyeva and Desmond Khor*
Department of Surgery, Texas Tech University Health Sciences Center, Lubbock, USA

*Address all correspondence to: desmond.khor@ttuhsc.edu

References

[1] Majano D. Workplace Injury & fatality statistics efsi.org: Electrical Safety Foundation International. 2025. Available from: https://www.esfi.org/workplace-safety/workplace-injury-fatality-statistics/ [Accessed: 2025-March-23]

[2] Lee RC. Injury by electrical forces: Pathophysiology, manifestations, and therapy. The Journal of Emergency Medicine. 1997;**34**(9):677–764

[3] Arnoldo BD, Purdue GF. The diagnosis and management of electrical injuries. Hand Clinics. 2009;**25**(4): 469–479

[4] Shih JG, Shahrokhi S, Jeschke MG. Review of Adult Electrical Burn Injury outcomes worldwide: An Analysis of Low-Voltage vs High-Voltage Electrical Injury. Journal of Burn Care & Research. 2017;**38**(1):e293–e8

[5] Khor D, AlQasas T, Galet C, Barrash J, Granchi T, Bertellotti R, et al. Electrical injuries and outcomes: A retrospective review. Burns 2023;**49**:1739–1744

[6] Zemaitis MR, Guirguis M, Cindass R. Electrical Injuries. Treasure Island (FL): StatPearls; 2025

[7] Saffle JR, Davis B, Williams P, Tabarp G. Recent outcomes in the Treatment of Burn Injury in the United States: A Report From the American burn association patient registry. Joumal of Bum Care & Rehabilitation. 1995;**16** (May/June 1995):219–32

[8] Dechent D, Emonds T, Stunder D, Schmiedchen K, Kraus T, Driessen S. Direct current electrical injuries: A systematic review of case reports and case series. Burns. 2020;**46**(2):267–278

[9] Bernal E, Arnoldo BD. 38 - Electrical Injuries. In: Herndon DN, editor. Total Burn Care. 5th ed. Edinburgh, London, New York, Oxford, Philadelphia, St Louis, Sydney: Elsevier; 2018. p. 396–402

[10] Gentges J, Schieche C. Electrical injuries in the emergency department: An evidence-based review. Emergency Medicine and Practice. 2018;**20**(11): 1–20

[11] Hunt JL, Mason Jr AD, Masterson TS, Pruitt Jr BA. The pathophysiology of acute electric injuries. The Journal of Trauma: Injury, Infection, and Critical Care. 1976;**16** (5):335–340

[12] Lee RC, Zhang D, Hannig J. Biophysical injury mechanisms in electrical shock trauma. Annual Review of Biomedical Engineering. 2000;**2**: 477–509

[13] Chen W, Lee RC. Evidence for electrical shock-induced conformational damage of voltage-gated ionic channels. Annals of the New York Academy of Sciences. 1994;**720**:124–135

[14] Zhang J, Qiao YR, Yang YD, Pan GZ, Lv CQ. Recovering from prolonged cardiac arrest induced by electric shock: A case report. World Journal of Clinical Cases. 2024;**12** (13):2248–2253

[15] Wesner ML, Hickie J. Long-term sequelae of electrical injury. Canadian Family Physician Medecin de Famille Canadien. 2013;**59**(9):935–939

[16] Koller J. High-tension electrical-arc-induced thermal burns caused by railway overhead cables. Burns. 1991;**17**(5):411–414

[17] Arnoldo B, Klein M, Gibran NS. Practice guidelines for the management of electrical injuries. Journal of Burn Care & Research. 2006;**27**(4):439–447

[18] Fish R. Electric shock, Part I: Physics and pathophysiology. The Journal of Emergency Medicine. 1993;**11** (3):309–312

[19] Orak M, Ustündağ M, Güloğlu C, Gökhan S, Alyan O. Relation between serum Pro-Brain natriuretic peptide, myoglobin, CK levels and morbidity and mortality in high voltage electrical injuries. Internal Medicine. 2010;**49** (22):2439–2443

[20] Fish R. Electric shock, Part II: Nature and mechanisms of injury. The Journal of Emergency Medicine. 1993;**11** (4):457–462

[21] Schneider JC, Qu HD. Neurologic and musculoskeletal complications of burn injuries. Physical Medicine and Rehabilitation Clinics of North America. 2011;**22**(2):261–275. vi

[22] Modayil PC, Lloyd GW, Mallik A, Bowdler DA. Inner ear damage following electric current and lightning injury: A literature review. European Archives of Oto-Rhino-Laryngology. 2014;**271**(5):855–861

[23] DiVincenti FC, Moncrief JA, Pruitt Jr BA. Electrical injuries: A review of 65 cases. The Journal of Trauma: Injury, Infection, and Critical Care. 1969;**9** (6):497–507

[24] Purdue GF, Arnoldo BD, Hunt JL. Chapter 39-Electrical injuries. In: Herndon DN, editor. Total Burn Care. 3th edn. Edinburgh: W.B. Saunders; 2007. p. 513–520

[25] Koumbourlis AC. Electrical injuries. Critical Care Medicine. 2002;**30**(11 Suppl):S424–30

[26] System JT. Clinical Practice guideline: Burn Care. 2025

[27] Fish RM, Geddes LA. Conduction of electrical current to and through the human body: A review. Eplasty. 2009;**9**:e44

[28] Beyene R. Electrical Injury Practice Management Guideline. Nashville, TN: Vanderbilt University Medical Center; 2022

[29] Culnan DM, Farner K, Bitz GH, Capek KD, Tu Y, Jimenez C, et al. Volume resuscitation in patients with high-voltage electrical injuries. Annals of Plastic Surgery 2018;**80**:S113–S8

[30] Kodadek L, Carmichael SP, Seshadri A, Pathak A, Hoth J, Appelbaum R, et al. Rhabdomyolysis: An American Association for the Surgery of Trauma Critical Care committee clinical consensus document. Trauma Surgery & Acute Care Open 2022;**7**:e000836

[31] Arnoldo BD, Purdue GF, Kowalske K, Helm PA, Burris A, Hunt JL. Electrical injuries: A 20-year review. The Journal of Burn Care & Rehabilitation. 2004;**25**(6):479–484

[32] Cooper MA. Lightning injuries: Prognostic signs for death. Annals of Emergency Medicine. 1980;**9**(3): 134–138

[33] Davis C, Engeln A, Johnson EL, McIntosh SE, Zafren K, Islas AA, et al.

Wilderness Medical Society practice guidelines for the prevention and treatment of lightning injuries: 2014 update. Wilderness & Environmental Medicine 2014;**25**:S86–95

[34] Hawkins E, Gostigian G, Diurba S. Lightning strike injuries. Emergency Medicine Clinics of North America. 2024;**42**(3):667–678

[35] van Ruler R, Eikendal T, Kooij FO, EC T. A shocking injury: A clinical review of lightning injuries highlighting pitfalls and a treatment protocol. Injury. 2022;**53**(10):3070–3077

[36] Cao D, Arens AM, Chow SL, Easter SR, Hoffman RS, Lagina AT, et al. Part 10: Adult and Pediatric special circumstances of Resuscitation: 2025 American Heart Association Guidelines for Cardiopulmonary Resuscitation and Emergency Cardiovascular Care. Circulation 2025;**152**:S578–S672

[37] Mutter E, Langley A. Cutaneous Lichtenberg figures from lightning strike. Canadian Medical Association Journal. 2019;**191**(9):E260. DOI: 10.1503/cmaj.181221

Section 4

Advanced Wound Healing and Regenerative Therapies

Chapter 7

Wound Healing with Modern Burn Dressing with a Focus on Synthetic Polylactic Acid Membrane as the Best Example

Mehmet Demircan, Kubilay Gürünlüoğlu, Tuğrul Çiçek and Necmettin Akpinar

Abstract

Burn injuries remain a significant global health concern, characterized by high morbidity and mortality rates. The management of burn wounds presents multifaceted challenges, including infection control, pain management, and the minimization of scar formation. While traditional dressing methods often fall short of meeting these clinical needs, the emergence of biomimetic and synthetic materials has shifted the treatment paradigm. This review examines the role of modern burn dressings in wound healing mechanisms, focusing specifically on Polylactic Acid Membrane (PLM) (Suprathel®), a synthetic lactide-caprolactone terpolymer. Literature evidence indicates that such synthetic membranes suppress bacterial colonization by optimizing moisture balance, triggering angiogenesis through lactate release, and creating a relatively acidic pH environment. The "Shift to Synthetics" process has just been very important in burn wound treatment. Clinical studies demonstrate that these modern synthetic dressings significantly reduce pain scores and shorten hospital stays compared to traditional silver dressings, particularly in the pediatric population. In conclusion, modern synthetic dressings offer a cost-effective alternative that accelerates regeneration and maximizes patient comfort without increasing the risk of infection. Synthetic skin substitutes have become not just an "aid" but an "active component" managing the healing process in burn surgery. As technological innovations increase, minimizing functional and aesthetic losses following burn injury will remain the ultimate goal.

Keywords: burn wound healing, modern burn dressing, polylactic acid membrane, synthetic skin substitute, pediatric burn

1. Introduction

Modern burn dressings are a rapidly developing and highly in-depth field in terms of regenerative medicine and biomaterials science [1, 2].

Burn injuries remain a significant global health concern, characterized by high morbidity and mortality rates [3]. Effective management requires a multifaceted approach that addresses infection control, fluid balance, and tissue regeneration [4]. Traditional dressings, such as silver sulfadiazine, while effective in antimicrobial activity, often hinder the visual assessment of the wound and can be associated with painful dressing changes. Consequently, there has been a paradigm shift toward modern biosynthetic dressings that mimic the natural extracellular matrix, thereby facilitating faster re-epithelialization and improving patient outcomes.

The healing process of a burn wound; hemostasis is a dynamic and complex biological phenomenon involving stages of inflammation, proliferation, and remodeling. As burn depth increases, the skin's barrier function is lost, and the body becomes susceptible to infections, excessive fluid loss, and hypothermia. Gauze and simple topical agents used in traditional treatment methods may be insufficient in protecting the wound from external factors and, most importantly, can delay healing by mechanically damaging newly formed granulation tissue during frequent dressing changes. Almost 70% of burn patients are at risk of developing hypertrophic scarring [5, 6]. Modern wound dressings have also reduced this rate. Due to the shortcomings of conventional dressings (gauze, etc.), there is a need for modern, intelligent dressings. Characteristic features that a modern dressing should possess include: maintaining moisture balance (moist environment), allowing gas exchange, controlling exudate, providing an antimicrobial barrier, painless dressing change, biocompatible and mimics the normal skin tissue. The biggest revolution in burn wound management in the last two decades has been the acceptance of the "moist wound healing" principle [7]). The "Moist Wound Healing" principle is crucial in modern literature. This principle advocates for a balance in the wound bed where it is neither too dry nor too wet [6]. Modern dressing technologies go beyond achieving this balance, offering smart materials that biochemically modulate the wound microenvironment, block pain at the receptor level, and act as a scaffold for epithelial cell migration. The "Shift to Synthetics" process has just been very important in burn wound treatment. While biological grafts (allografts or xenografts) were popular in the past, today products like Polylactic acid membrane (PLM)(=Suprathel®) are preferred due to their lack of immunological response and logistical ease (ability to be stored at room temperature) [8]. This review examines the evolution of modern burn dressings, focusing particularly on the clinical efficacy of PLM, representing the cutting edge of synthetic polymer technology, and their comparative analysis with traditional methods. Furthermore, this section will address particularly in the treatment of second-degree (superficial and deep dermal) partial burns and in closing donor sites from which skin grafts have been taken in pediatric use, as the most common age group for burn injuries is children aged 0-5 years with scald burns.

2. Simply classification of modern dressing technologies

We can classified of modern burn dressings as follow [1, 2]

- Hydrogels and Hydrocolloids: High water content and cooling effect.
- Alginates: Seaweed-derived materials for managing dense exudate.
- Films and Foams: Permeability and cushioning properties.

- Biological and Biosynthetic Dressings: Collagen-based structures and skin graft substitutes.
- Nanotechnology Dressings: Silver nanoparticles (AgNPs) or systems with controlled drug release.
- Synthetic and Biodegradable Skin Substitutes: Polylactic acid membrane (PLM)
- Smart and Active Dressings (Emerging Technologies)
- Bioactive Dressings: Systems containing growth factors (EGF, VEGF) or stem cells.
- Smart Sensors: Dressings that detect infection with changes in pH, temperature, or humidity.
- 3D Bio-printing: Personalized "skin" scaffolds.

3. Focusing on synthetic PLM as the best example of modern burn dressings

In actual burn wound treatment, it's necessary to mention the concept of "Shift to Synthetics"[9]. While biological grafts (allografts/xenografts) were popular in the past, it's important to emphasize that products like PLM are now preferred due to their lack of immunological response and ease of logistics (being able to be stored at room temperature). Fully synthetic and absorbable, biodegradable skin substitutes, such as PLM, which act like a biological dressing without the risks of infection or rejection associated with biological materials (e.g., cadaver skin or pig-derived products), are of critical importance [10–13].

Taking PLM as an example of "Synthetic and Biodegradable Skin Substitutes"; it is a fully synthetic membrane that is becoming the gold standard, particularly in the treatment of second-degree partial burns and in closing donor sites.

Burn management involves multifaceted challenges such as regulation of inflammatory process, infection control, pain management, and scarring. While traditional dressings often fall short, modern synthetic dressings like PLM offer a **biomimetic** approach. This review examines how this membrane optimize the wound environment by inducing angiogenesis, regulating oxidative stress molecules and providing a bacterial barrier through wound's pH modulation. There are a lot of clinical and experimental evidences show significant reduction in pain scores and hospitalization time, particularly in pediatric patients [14–29].

3.1 Structure and composition

- Material: PLM is a "Lacto-capromer" terpolymer. It contains Polylactic acid, trimethylene carbonate, and epsilon-caprolactone (Lacto-capromer).
- Biocompatibility: Being completely synthetic, there is no risk of transmission of animal or human-derived diseases, eliminating religious/ethical concerns.

- Failure in the Body: While remaining on the wound, it is broken down over time through hydrolysis and excreted from the body only as CO_2 and H_2O.

3.2 Mechanism of action (why is it called "second skin"?)

- The most important feature that distinguishes PLM from classic dressings is that it mimics the physical properties of human skin (elasticity, water vapor permeability)

- The effects on stasis zone: The effects of PLM on stasis zones is well studied by clinically and experimentally. It modulates oxidative status by decreasing oxidative stress factors and increasing anti-oxidative factors, either locally or systematically [18–21].

- Pain management: When applied to the wound surface, it immediately isolates nerve endings. Clinical studies show that it provides up to a 60% reduction in pain, as well as reducing the need for analgesic use [26].

- pH balance: During healing, it modulates the pH of the wound decreasing alkaline value. The modulated pH of the environment suppresses bacterial growth and accelerates epithelialization.

- Transparency: It becomes transparent after application; this allows the doctor to monitor the underlying healing process and signs of infection without removing the dressing.

3.3 Advantages of PLM use

- Single application: After cleaning and/or debridement of burn wound, it can be applied once and remains on the wound until healing is complete (average 10-14 days). As the wound heals, it dries and flakes off on its own as you can see easily.

- Scar control: By shortening the healing process, preventing damage to the granulation tissue from constant dressing changes, and regulating factors such as TGF-β3 in the scar tissue, it reduces the risk of hypertrophic scar formation [5, 13, 18, 30, 31].

If we look at the most current clinical data regarding the administration protocol and pediatric use of PLM;

3.4 PLM application protocol (step-by-step)

The key to success in clinical trials is the complete adaptation of the dressing to the wound. The protocol generally consists of the following steps:

- Wound preparation (Critical stage): The wound should be cleaned with sterile solutions and necrotic tissues should be completely removed. Especially in children, the use of hydro-surgery is recommended to prepare a viable and bleeding wound bed to which PLM can adhere [27, 32, 33].

- Hemostasis: Bleeding must be completely stopped before application (with warm compresses and/or adrenaline pads). Blood accumulation may cause the dressing to detach from the wound bed and lead to infection.

- Application: The membrane is placed so that it extends approximately 1 cm beyond the wound margins. Softening it with body heat (by warming it between the hands) increases adaptation to the wound.

- Fixation and layering: Usually does not require sutures; however, in children or in mobile areas (joints), it can be fixed with a single suture or staple. A paraffin or oil-based gauze and dressing must be applied over the wound.

- Follow-up: External dressings (gauze) are changed every 3–5 days depending on the amount of exudation, but PLM should never be removed from the wound. As epithelialization is complete (usually on days 10–14), the dressing dries and detaches from the skin on its own [18].

3.5 Use and advantages in pediatric burns

Ten-year retrospective studies and randomized controlled trials on the use of PLM in pediatric patients highlight the following results [10–11, 14–30]:

- Pain management: Studies show that children in PLM group have significantly lower pain scores (COMFORT-B or VAS) during dressing changes and at rest compared to traditional dressings (e.g., Mepilex Ag) [34–39].

- Hospital stay: The median hospital stay in pediatric patients is reduced to 4–5 days with PLM. This allows children to return to their social environment more quickly.

- Reduced graft needs: Even in deep dermal (degree 2) burns, the use of PLM reduces the rate of surgical grafting (skin transplantation) by approximately 20-30%.

- Scar quality: According to POSAS and Vancouver Scar Scale results, children treated with PLM showed higher scar elasticity and fewer pigmentation abnormalities at 6 and 12-month follow-ups.

3.6 Key clinical and experimental findings

- Healing speed and epithelialization: The median healing time in pediatric cases is between 12.5 and 13 days. Although this period can extend up to 29 days in wounds that develop infection or colonize, the overall risk of infection is not higher than with traditional dressings [18–21].

- Microbiology: The most common pathogen is Staphylococcus aureus. PML's ability to create a slightly acidic pH (with lactic acid release) forms a barrier that naturally suppresses bacterial proliferation in the wound bed [40].

- Cost-effectiveness: Although the unit price of the product is high, it has been reported that the total treatment cost is lower due to the reduction in the number of dressing changes, the decrease in the need for anesthesia/sedation, and the shortening of the hospital stay.
- The biggest advantage of PLM is that it minimizes the anxiety or psychological trauma associated with dressing changes seen in the pediatric population.

PLM's mechanism of action is described in the literature not only as a physical barrier but also as an active system that biochemically modulates the wound microenvironment. In literature, this is often referred to as a "biomimetic" approach. In light of the findings in the literature, we can detail PLM's main mechanisms of action on healing under the following headings:

3.6.1 Dynamic moisture and gas permeability

PLM is designed to mimic the transepidermal water loss (TEWL) of human skin [7].

- Vapor permeability: Due to its structure, it initially has high vapor permeability. It allows the removal of excess exudate (fluid) from the wound surface while preventing desiccation of the wound.
- Wound bed balance: When the ideal moisture balance is achieved, the migration of keratinocytes over the wound surface (lateral migration) is accelerated.

3.6.2 Lactate production and pH modulation

When PLM is broken down through hydrolysis, it slowly releases lactic acid into the environment. The literature states that this process has two critical effects:

- Antimicrobial environment: The release of lactic acid lowers the pH value at the wound surface (acidic environment). Most pathogenic bacteria (especially Pseudomonas aeruginosa and Staphylococcus aureus) prefer alkaline environments. Acidic pH inhibits the proliferation of these bacteria.
- Angiogenesis stimulation: Increased lactate concentration in the wound bed stimulates the release of VEGF (Vascular Endothelial Growth Factor) by macrophages. This accelerates neovascularization, increasing tissue nutrition.

3.6.3 Nociceptive (pain) mechanism

In studies on modern dressings, PLM's pain relief mechanism is explained by "nerve end isolation":

- Isolation Effect: When the membrane adheres tightly to the wound bed (adhesion), it cuts off contact between exposed nerve endings and airflow and external stimuli [17].
- Inflammation Control: By stabilizing the levels of inflammatory cytokines (IL-1, IL-6) on wound bed and into stasis zone, it prevents overstimulation of pain-sensitive nociceptors [18–21].

3.6.4 Biomechanical adaptation and prevention of contact inhibition

PLMI's physical structure is in mechanical compatibility with biological systems:

- Plasticity: When heated, it adapts to all the folds (micro-indentations) of the wound. This prevents the formation of "dead space" on the wound and reduces the risk of bacterial colonization due to fluid accumulation.

- Keratinocyte migration: Its synthetic structure acts as a scaffold for epithelial cells (keratinocytes) to adhere to and migrate. As epithelial cells migrate under the covering, PLM rises upwards, thus preventing mechanical damage to the newly formed tissue.

3.6.5 Cost-effectiveness paradox

Many randomized controlled trials in the literature emphasize that although PLM has a higher unit cost, it is more advantageous in terms of total treatment cost (including hospital stay) because it reduces the number of secondary dressing changes and lowers the need for narcotic analgesics [26, 27].

3.7 Comparison of PLM vs. Silver-based dressings

3.7.1 Mechanistic comparison

In modern burn treatment, PLM and silver dressings (antimicrobial barriers) operate with different philosophies. Silver dressings focus more on "preventing and clearing infection," while PLM focuses on "promoting regeneration and stabilizing the wound bed." The **Table 1** provides a summary to compare these two technologies at a mechanistic level [18–20, 34–36.

- Cell proliferation: While the literature indicates that long-term use of silver ions can sometimes delay wound healing (re-epithelialization) (cytotoxic effect), PLM emphasizes that it supports fibroblast activity and collagen synthesis thanks to lactate release.

- Psychological Factors: Especially in pediatric cases, the periodic changes of silver dressings can cause anxiety and pain in children, while PLM's "apply and forget" principle maximizes treatment compliance.

- Cost: The unit cost of silver dressings is low, but frequent changes, additional consumables, and personnel time increase costs. With PLM, the product cost is high, while the operational cost is low.

3.7.2 Evidence-based comparison

Clinical studies comparing PLM and silver dressings (especially Acticoat or Mepilex Ag) provide very strong evidence in the literature regarding "Evidence-Based Medicine". The most striking case analyses and clinical study results are as follows (**Tables 2, 3**):

Features	**PLM**	**Silver Dressings**
Key Function	Biomimetic "Second Skin" and Scaffold	Broad-spectrum Antimicrobial Barrier
Mechanism of Action	pH reduction (lactic acid), triggering angiogenesis	Bacterial DNA/enzyme degradation with silver ions
Wound Bed pH	Acidic: Suppresses bacterial growth, stimulates epithelialization	Neutral/Alkaline: The effectiveness of silver may vary depending on pH
Dressing Change	Single application; remains on the wound until heal	Requires frequent changes every 3–7 days (depending on the product)
Pain Control	Very High: Completely isolates nerve endings	Moderate: Trauma/pain may occur during dressing change
Cytotoxicity	None; It has a cell-friendly structure.	It can be toxic to keratinocytes and fibroblasts in high concentrations.
Transparency	It is transparent; the wound bed can be directly observed	It is usually opaque/dark colored; it needs to be opened for wound monitoring
Infection Management	Provides a barrier and suppresses pH; not recommended in active infection	Effective in fighting active infection and high colonization
Clinical Use	Clean, debrided 2nd degree burns especially first two days	Contaminated or high-risk wounds for infection, especially late 2nd degree burns.

Table 1.
Comparison of PLM vs. Silver dressings.

Parameter	**PLM**	**Silver Dressings**	**P Value (Significance)**
Mean Pain Score (VAS 1-10)	1.8 – 2.4	3.5 – 5.1	$p < 0.001$ (Highly significant)
Complete Epithelialization Time (Days)	12.3 ± 2.1	13.9 ± 3.4	$p > 0.05$ (Similar)
Number of Dressing Changes (14 days)	1 – 2 times (Outer layer only)	4 – 7 times (Complete change)	$p < 0.001$
Infection Rate (%)	2.4	2.1	$p > 0.05$ (Clinically equal)
Hospital Stay (Days)	7.4 ± 1.5	9.2 ± 2.8	$p < 0.05$

Table 2.
PLM and silver dressings (nano-crystalline silver) – clinical data comparison.

3.7.2.1 Comparative study on pediatric scalding burns

PLM provides an optimal micro-environment for the treatment of partial-thickness burns in children [26].

- Case Group: Children with second-degree (partial-thickness) burns.
- Comparison: PLM versus traditional silver dressings and xenografts (pig skin).
- Findings: * Pain Score: Pain scores from the first 24 hours of dressing application were significantly lower in children using PLM compared to the silver dressing group.

Author/Year	Patient Group (n)	Burn Type	Key Outcome
Schwarze et al. [26]	n = 22 (Pediatric)	2. Degree (Scald)	A 60% reduction in pain scores and rapid epithelialization were observed in the PLM group
Schwarze et al. [27]	n = 30	2. Degree Deep	The excellent adaptation of the synthetic membrane to the wound bed and the advantage of easy application were emphasized
Uhlig et al. [36]	n = 40 (Split-body)	2. Degree Partial	Equality in infection control; significant difference in patient comfort and nursing workload in favor of PLM
Rashaan et al. [17]	Systematic Review	Pediatric Burns	PLM was concluded to be a candidate for the "gold standard" in children and to be cost-effective
Hundeshagen [34]	n = 124	Pediatric	The need for secondary surgery (grafting) was 15-20% lower in the PLM group.

Table 3.
Summary of key studies in the literature (evidence table).

- o Healing Time: Complete epithelialization was achieved in an average of 12–13 days.
- o Conclusion: The authors emphasized that PLM reduced "dressing change trauma" to almost zero in children.

3.7.2.2 Competing with the gold standard: PLM vs. Nanocrystalline silver dressings

PLM vs. nanocrystalline silver dressings in the treatment of partial-thickness burns [36]:

Method: Two similar burn areas on the patients' bodies were selected (split-body study); PLM was applied to one area and nanocrystalline silver dressing to the other.

Findings:

- Infection Rate: No significant difference was found in terms of infection between the two groups. This showed that PLM, despite not containing silver, was as protective as silver thanks to its acidic pH barrier.
- Comfort: Patients reported that the area where PLM was applied was much more flexible and they did not feel "stretching/pulling" while moving.
- Cost: It was calculated that the nursing care time was 40% less in the PLM group thanks to the single application.

3.7.2.3 Epithelialization dynamics in deep dermal burns

It was observed that silver dressings could cause a "staining" effect (silver staining/toxicity) that slowed healing in some cases, while in cases where PLM was applied, epithelialization in the form of "islands" started earlier due to the effect of lactate and regulating oxidative stress, locally and systematically [18–21]. It was noted that because PLM's transparent structure allowed healing islands to be seen, surgeons could avoid unnecessary grafting operations.

Case series in the literature demonstrate that modern synthetic PLM provide non-inferior infection control compared to antimicrobial silver dressings. However, it's main advantage lies in its biomimetic structure, which dramatically reduces nociceptive pain and minimizes the need for surgical sedation in pediatric patients [26, 27, 36].

3.7.2.4 An easy "clinical decision algorithm proposal"

1. Is the wound clean and in the early stages (first 48 hours)? → PLM (Maximum regeneration and pain control).

2. Is the wound contaminated or is there suspicion of infection? → Silver based dressings (Antimicrobial efficacy is prioritized).

3. Is the wound very deep (grade 3) and wide? → Dermal scaffolds (Integra, Matriderm, or Synthetic matrices etc.) + auto grafting.

4. Discussion

The clinical efficacy of PLM is largely attributed to its unique biochemical properties. Upon application, the degradation of the polylactic acid component leads to a sustained release of lactate into the wound microenvironment. This acidic shift not only exerts a bacteriostatic effect but also serves as a potent stimulus for angiogenesis and fibroblast proliferation. Furthermore, the semi-permeable nature of the membrane ensures an optimal moisture balance, preventing wound desiccation while allowing for gaseous exchange. Our clinical observations, consistent with the literature, suggest that the reduction in dressing change frequency significantly lowers the physiological stress and pain experienced by pediatric patients.

The fundamental goal in modern burn management is to promote rapid epithelialization without traumatizing the wound bed. The data examined in this study prove that synthetic membranes such as PLM are a strong competitor to traditional silver (nanocrystalline silver) dressings. Comparative studies have shown that despite the known antimicrobial power of silver, the acidic microenvironment created by PLM also provides similar infection control. However, the main point of divergence between these two technologies is the dynamics of cell comfort and tissue regeneration.

While the potential cytotoxic effects of silver ions continue to be debated in the literature, the release of lactate through hydrolysis of PLM directly supports angiogenesis by stimulating macrophage activity and vascular endothelial growth factor (VEGF) expression [17–20]. Especially in pediatric cases, as highlighted. The 'painless dressing' phenomenon not only improves the patient's quality of life but also reduces the need for repeated sedation, thereby lowering the risk of systemic complications [26].

Although cost analyses show the high unit price of the product, the reduction in dressing change frequency and shorter hospital stays prove that modern synthetics are also economically sustainable [34]. Future studies should focus on combining these synthetic scaffolds with growth factors or stem cells to transform them into a "smart dressing" form.

5. Conclusion and future perspectives

5.1 Conclusion

In conclusion, modern synthetic dressings, exemplified by Polylactic Acid Membranes, represent a transformative advancement in burn care. By integrating biomimetic properties with superior clinical handling, these materials offer an optimal environment for wound healing. They not only accelerate the recovery process but also significantly enhance the quality of life for patients by minimizing pain and reducing the need for invasive procedures. As the field of regenerative medicine evolves, the integration of these synthetic scaffolds into standard burn protocols is expected to become the gold standard, particularly in specialized pediatric burn units.

5.2 Future perspectives

The future of burn treatment lies in the integration of "smart" and "personalized" technologies. The following developments are expected to come to the forefront in the next decade:

- Smart Sensor Integration: Thanks to nanosensors embedded in existing synthetic dressings, the pH, temperature, and humidity of the wound can be monitored instantly via smartphones, and infection can be diagnosed before clinical symptoms appear [2].

- 3D Bio-printing: The goal is to produce patient-specific skin equivalents in the operating room by printing "living inks" obtained from the patient's own cells (keratinocytes and fibroblasts) onto synthetic scaffolds similar to PLM [1, 2].

- Growth Factor and Drug Release: Experimental studies are ongoing on doubling the healing rate with controlled-release growth factors (EGF, TGF-beta) or exophytic agents encapsulated within polymer structures [1, 2, 13].

As a result, synthetic skin substitutes have become not just an "aid" but an "active component" managing the healing process in burn surgery. As technological innovations increase, minimizing functional and aesthetic losses following burn injury will remain the ultimate goal.

Acknowledgements

The authors acknowledge the use of ChatGPT for language editing in the chapter.

Author details

Mehmet Demircan*, Kubilay Gürünlüoğlu, Tuğrul Çiçek and Necmettin Akpinar
Department of Pediatric Surgery and Pediatric Burn Center, İnönü University School of Medicine, Malatya, Türkiye

*Address all correspondence to: mehmet.demircan@inonu.edu.tr

References

[1] Queen D, Orsted H, Sanada H, Sussman G. A dressing history. International Wound Journal. 2004;**1** (1):59–77. DOI: 10.1111/j.1742-4801.2004.0009.x

[2] Rezvani Ghomi E, Niazi M, Ramakrishna S. The evolution of wound dressings: From traditional to smart dressings. Polymers for Advanced Technologies. 2023;**34**(2):520–530. DOI: 10.1093/jbcr/iraf143

[3] Lee N, Bae Y, Jang S, Lee DW, Lee SW. Global, regional, and national burden of burn injury by total body surface area (TBSA) involvement from 1990 to 2021, with Projections of Prevalence to 2050. Healthcare (Basel). 2025;**13**(16):2077. DOI: 10.3390/healthcare13162077

[4] Cretu A, Grosu-Bularda A, Bordeanu-Diaconescu E-M, Hodea F-V, Ratoiu V-A, Dumitru C-S, Andrei M-C, Neagu T-P, Lascar I, Hariga C-S. Strategies for Optimizing Acute Burn Wound Therapy: A Comprehensive Review. Medicina (Kaunas). 2025;**61**(1):128. DOI: 10.3390/medicina61010128

[5] Finnerty CC, Jeschke MG, Branski LK, Barret JP, Dziewulski P, Herndon DN. Hypertrophic scarring: The greatest unmet challenge after burn injury. The Lancet. 2016;**388**:1427–1436. DOI: 10.1016/S0140-6736(16)31406-4

[6] Nabai L, Pourghadiri A, Ghahary A. Hypertrophic scarring: Current knowledge of predisposing factors, cellular and molecular mechanisms. Journal of Burn Care & Research: Official Publication of the American Burn Association. 2020;**41**(1):48–56. DOI: 10.1093/jbcr/irz158

[7] Winter GD. Formation of the scab and the rate of epithelization of superficial wounds in the skin of the young domestic pig. Nature. 1962;**20** (193):293–294. DOI: 10.1038/193293a0

[8] Świerczyńska M, Kudzin MH, Chruściel JJ. Poly(lactide)-Based Materials Modified with Biomolecules: A Review. Materials (Basel, Switzerland). 2024;**17** (21):5184. DOI: 10.3390/ma17215184

[9] Horn CP, Fierro AL, Lantis JC. The shift to synthetics: A review of novel synthetic matrices for wound closure. Surgical Technology International. 2023;**42**:75–86

[10] van de Warenburg MS, El Yadari S, Hummelink S, Ulrich DJ, Vehmeijer-Heeman M. Suprathel's usability and effectiveness for the treatment of paediatric partial thickness burns: A 10-year retrospective cohort study. Burns. 2025;**51**(4):107451. DOI: 10.1016/j.burns.2025.107451

[11] Blome-Eberwein SA, Amani H, Lozano DD, Gogal C, Boorse D, Pagella P. A bio-degradable synthetic membrane to treat superficial and deep second degree burn wounds in adults and children – 4 year experience. Burns. 2021;**47**(4):838–846. DOI: 10.1016/j.burns.2020.08.008

[12] Afnan MAM, Saxena AK. Tissue repair in neonatal and paediatric surgery: Analysis of infection in surgical implantation of synthetic resorbable biomaterials. Bio-medical Materials and Engineering. 2018;**29**(6):799–808. DOI: 10.3233/BME-181024

[13] Jeschke MG, van Baar ME, Choudhry MA, Chung KK, Gibran NS, Logsetty S. Burn injury. Nature Reviews

Disease Primers. 2020;**6**:11. DOI: 10.1038/s41572-020-0145-5

[14] Nguyen AT, Chikoti R, Bell D. Polylactic acid skin substitute in pediatric burn management: A systematic literature review and meta-analysis. Journal of Burn Care & Research. 2026;**47**(1):236–245. DOI: 10.1093/jbcr/iraf143

[15] Delgado-Miguel C, García Morán A, Fuentes Gómez L, Díaz M, Miguel-Ferrero M, López-Gutiérrez JC. Comparison of the effectiveness of three different skin substitutes for the treatment of pediatric burns. European Journal of Pediatrics. 2024;**184**(1):80. DOI: 10.1007/s00431-024-05916-6

[16] Raine BE, Fowler CC, Nguyen A, Schneider P, Gunn KJ, Chikoti R, Bell DE. Polylactic acid membrane for the treatment of pediatric burn injuries: An adoptable practice to improve burn management. Annals of Plastic Surgery. 2025;**94**(Suppl 4):S218–S222. DOI: 10.1016/j.burns.2020.08.008

[17] Rashaan ZM, Krijnen P, Allema JH, Vloemans AF, Schipper IB, Breederveld RS. Usability and effectiveness of Suprathel® in partial thickness burns in children. European Journal of Trauma and Emergency Surgery. 2017;**43**(4):549–556. DOI: 10.1007/s00068-016-0708-z

[18] Demircan M, Gürünlüoğlu K, Gözükara Bağ HG, Koçbıyık A, Gül M, Üremiş N, Gül S, Gürünlüoğlu S, Türköz Y, Taşçı A. Impaction of the polylactic membrane or hydrofiber with silver dressings on the interleukin-6, tumor necrosis factor-α, transforming growth factor-b3 levels in the blood and tissues of pediatric patients with burns. Ulusal Travma Ve Acil Cerrahi Dergisi = Turkish Journal of Trauma & Emergency Surgery: TJTES. 2021;**27**(1):122–131. DOI: 10.14744/tjtes.2020.30483

[19] Gürünlüoğlu K, Demircan M, Koç A, Koçbıyık A, Taşçı A, Durmuş K, Gürünlüoğlu S, Gözükara Bağ H. The Effects of Different Burn Dressings on Length of Telomere and Expression of Telomerase in Children With Thermal Burns. Journal of Burn Care & Research. 2019;**40**(3):302–311. DOI: 10.1093/jbcr/irz019

[20] Gürünlüoğlu K, Demircan M, Taşçı A, Üremiş MM, Türköz Y, Bağ HG, Akıncı A, Bayrakçı E. The Effects of Two Different Burn Dressings on Serum Oxidative Stress Indicators in Children with Partial Burn. Journal of Burn Care & Research. 2019;**40**(4):444–450. DOI: 10.1093/jbcr/irz037

[21] Haller HL, Sander F, Popp D, Rapp M, Hartmann B, Demircan M, Nischwitz SP, Kamolz LP. Oxygen, pH, Lactate, and Metabolism—How Old Knowledge and New Insights Might Be Combined for New Wound Treatment. Medicina (Kaunas). 2021;**57**(11):1190. DOI: 10.3390/medicina57111190

[22] Everett M, Massand S, Davis W, Burkey B, Glat PM. Use of a copolymer dressing on superficial and partial-thickness burns in a paediatric population. Journal of Wound Care. 2015;**24**(Sup7):S4–8. DOI: 10.12968/jowc.2015.24.Sup7.S4

[23] Fernandes S, Teixeira I, Carmo L, Campos M, Garcia M. The Use of a Polylactic Membrane in Pediatric Burns Proves to be Successful Even After Late Application. Journal of Burn Care & Research. 2023;**44**(5):1176–1181. DOI: 10.1093/jbcr/irad015

[24] Gögele C, Schulze-Tanzil G, Kokozidou M, Gäbel C, Billner M, Reichert B, Bodenschatz K. Growth characteristics of human juvenile, adult and murine fibroblasts: A comparison of polymer wound dressings. Journal of Wound Care. 2020;**29**(10):572–585. DOI: 10.12968/jowc.2020.29.10.572

[25] Highton L, Wallace C, Shah M. Use of Suprathel® for partial thickness burns in children. Burns. 2013;**39**(1):136–141. DOI: 10.1016/j.burns.2012.05.005

[26] Schwarze H, Küntscher M, Uhlig C, Hierlemann H, Prantl L, Noack N, Hartmann B. Suprathel®, a new skin substitute, in the management of donor sites of split-thickness skin grafts: Results of a clinical study. Burns. 2007;**33**(7):850–854. DOI: 10.1016/j.burns.2006.10.393

[27] Schwarze H, Küntscher MV, Uhlig C, Hierlemann H, Prantl L, Ottomann C, Hartmann B. Suprathel, a New Skin Substitute, in the Management of Partial-Thickness Burn Wounds: Results of a Clinical Study. Annals of Plastic Surgery. 2008;**60**:181–185. DOI: 10.1097/SAP.0b013e318056bbf6

[28] Raine BE, Fowler CC, Nguyen A, Schneider P, Gunn KJ, Chikoti R, Bell DE. Polylactic Acid Membrane for the Treatment of Pediatric Burn Injuries: An Adoptable Practice to Improve Burn Management. Annals of Plastic Surgery. 2025;**94**(Suppl 4S): S218–S222. DOI: 10.1097/SAP.0000000000004261

[29] Wachenfeld-Teschner V, Beier JP, Boos AM, Schäfer B. Factors Influencing Surgical Care and Outcome of Pediatric Burn Injuries and the Use of Synthetic Skin Substitutes. Journal of Burn Care & Research. 2025;**46**(1): 94–100. DOI: 10.1093/jbcr/irae106

[30] Vinaik R, Fish J, Jeschke MG. Burn Hypertrophic Scar in Pediatric Patients: Clinical Case. In Téot L, Mustoe TA, Middelkoop E, Gauglitz GG, Eds. Textbook on Scar Management: State of the Art Management and Emerging Technologies [Internet]. Cham (CH): Springer; 2020. DOI: 10.1007/978-3-030-44766-3_60

[31] Chiang RS, Borovikova AA, King K, Banyard DA, Lalezari S, Toranto JD, Paydar KZ, Wirth GA, Evans GR, Widgerow AD. Current concepts related to hypertrophic scarring in burn injuries. Wound Repair and Regeneration. 2016;**24**(3):466–477. DOI: 10.1111/wrr.12432

[32] Zhang Y, Guo K, Tian C, Tong L, Hu D, Wang Y. Limited debridement combined with ReCell® Techniques for deep second-degree burns. Journal of Plastic Surgery and Hand Surgery. 2024;**59**:72–76. DOI: 10.2340/jphs.v59.24557

[33] Schulz A, Perbix W, Shoham Y, Daali S, Charalampaki C, Fuchs PC, Schiefer J. Our initial learning curve in the enzymatic debridement of severely burned hands—Management and pit falls of initial treatments and our development of a post debridement wound treatment algorithm. Burns. 2017;**43**(2):326–336. DOI: 10.1016/j.burns.2016.08.009

[34] Hundeshagen G, Collins VN, Wurzer P, Sherman W, Voigt CD, Cambiaso-Daniel J, Nunez Lopez O, Sheaffer J, Herndon DN, Finnerty CC, Branski LK. A Prospective, Randomized, Controlled Trial Comparing the Outpatient Treatment of Pediatric and Adult Partial-Thickness

Burns with Suprathel or Mepilex Ag. Journal of Burn Care & Research. 2018;**39**(2):261–267. DOI: 10.1097/BCR.0000000000000584

[35] Karlsson M, Steinvall I, Elmasry M. Suprathel® or Mepilex® Ag for treatment of partial thickness burns in children: A case control study. Burns. 2023;**49**(7):1585–1591. DOI: 10.1016/j.burns.2023.03.003

[36] Uhlig C, Rapp M, Hartmann B, Hierlemann H, Planck H, Dittel -K-K. Suprathel®—An innovative, resorbable skin substitute for the treatment of burn victims. Burns. 2007;**33**(2):221–229. DOI: 10.1016/j.burns.2006.04.024

[37] Pardesi O, Fuzaylov G. Pain Management in Pediatric Burn Patients: Review of Recent Literature and Future Directions. Journal of Burn Care & Research. 2017;**38**(6):335–347. DOI: 10.1097/BCR.0000000000000470

[38] Ciornei B, David VL, Popescu D, Boia ES. Pain Management in Pediatric Burns: A Review of the Science behind It. Global Health, Epidemiology and Genomics. 2023;**2023**:9950870. DOI: 10.1155/2023/9950870

[39] Delgado DA, Lambert BS, Boutris N, McCulloch PC, Robbins AB, Moreno MR, Harris JD. Validation of Digital Visual Analog Scale Pain Scoring With a Traditional Paper-based Visual Analog Scale in Adults. Journal of the American Academy of Orthopaedic Surgeons. Global Research & Reviews. 2018;**2**(3):e088. DOI: 10.5435/JAAOSGlobal-D-17-00088

[40] Roy S, Mukherjee P, Kundu S, Majumder D, Raychaudhuri V, Choudhury L. Microbial infections in burn patients. Acute and Critical Care. 2024;**39**(2):214–225. DOI: 10.4266/acc.2023.01571

Chapter 8

Using Photobiomodulation in Treating Burn Ulcers

Nooshafarin Kazemikhoo and Chow A.M. Roberta

Abstract

Burns are the most frequent and distressing form of trauma. Despite the availability of standard treatments, the exploration of novel therapeutic strategies remains essential for advancing burn wound care. Photo biomodulation (PBM) has been used to treat acute and chronic wounds, including burns, diabetic ulcers, surgical wounds, pressure ulcers, and venous ulcers. PBM has anti-inflammatory effects, stimulates cellular activity, promotes tissue regeneration, induces the proliferation of follicular stem cells and follicular angiogenesis, and improves blood circulation.

Keywords: photo biomodulation, low-level laser therapy, cold laser, wound healing, burn ulcers

1. Introduction

Burns are common types of skin injuries encountered at all levels of medical facilities. Minor burns may heal with topical treatment alone, but moderate to severe burns might require systemic management and skin grafting. Delayed or inappropriate initial treatment might affect the prognosis. Burn injuries are associated with significant mortality and morbidity due to infections and scar formations [1].

Photo biomodulation (PBM) is one of the options to treat burn ulcers, especially the severe and complicated ones.

This chapter presents our insights drawn from more than 20 years of clinical experience in the treatment of different types of acute and chronic wounds, including burn ulcers, using PBM.

2. Clinical insights into managing burn ulcers, two decades of experience

Severe thermal tissue damage induces prominent inflammation in burn wounds compared to other types of wounds, and the persistent underlying inflammation dramatically delays the normal sequence of healing. Neutrophils, macrophages, and lymphocytes initiate the inflammatory phase, the classic clinical signs of which are redness, warmth, swelling, and pain in the affected area. Transforming growth factors-β (TGF-β), platelet-derived growth factor (PDGF), vascular endothelial growth factor (VEGF), and fibroblast growth factors (FGFs) play key roles in specific phases. The central wound healing cytokine is TGF-β, which affects different cell types involved in wound healing responses, including cell migration and infiltration, angiogenesis, matrix synthesis, and remodeling [1].

PBM, or low-level laser therapy, is an effective method for treating acute and chronic wounds, supported by several reviews and meta-analyses. It seems that PBM affects all the stages of inflammation, including early inflammation (Phase 1), repair and regeneration (Phase 2), and remodeling and maturation (Phase 3) [2, 3]. Myofibroblast-mediated matrix synthesis induces wound contraction during normal healing, although the persistence of these cells has been correlated with burn wound scarring and contractures. It seems that PBM can increase myofibroblast transformation, predominantly down-regulate the cytokine-cytokine receptor interaction pathway genes and some of the TGF-β signaling genes, independent of the TGF-β1/Smad pathway [4]. Our previous in-vivo study demonstrated the regulatory effects of PBM on FGF, PDGF, and VEGF expression at the mRNA level in diabetic and nondiabetic mice fibroblasts [5], and less scar or scarless healing in grades 2 and 3 burn ulcers in children [6] (**Figures 1–4**).

Macrophages clear debris and prevent infections, which play crucial roles in burn wound healing. PBM accelerates macrophage migration and phagocytic activity, and this chemotactic infiltration plays an important role in initiating resolution and wound clearance [7].

Epithelization is a main aspect of successful wound healing. Keratinocytes and growth factors play key roles in this process. TGF-βs, as latent secreted complexes, can be activated by light. TGF-βs promote proliferation and migration in a wide range of cell types [8] (**Figures 5–7**).

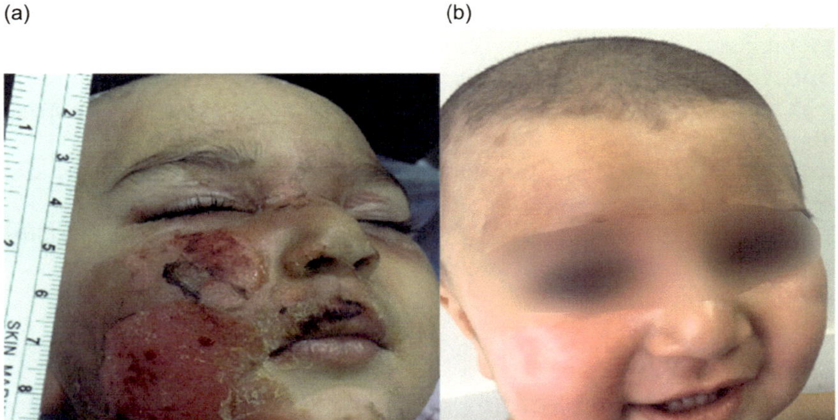

Figure 1.
(a) Grade 2b burn ulcer in an 8-month-old boy present for 2 days before treatment, (b) After 10 sessions of PBM using 650 nm red laser, $1 j/cm^2$.

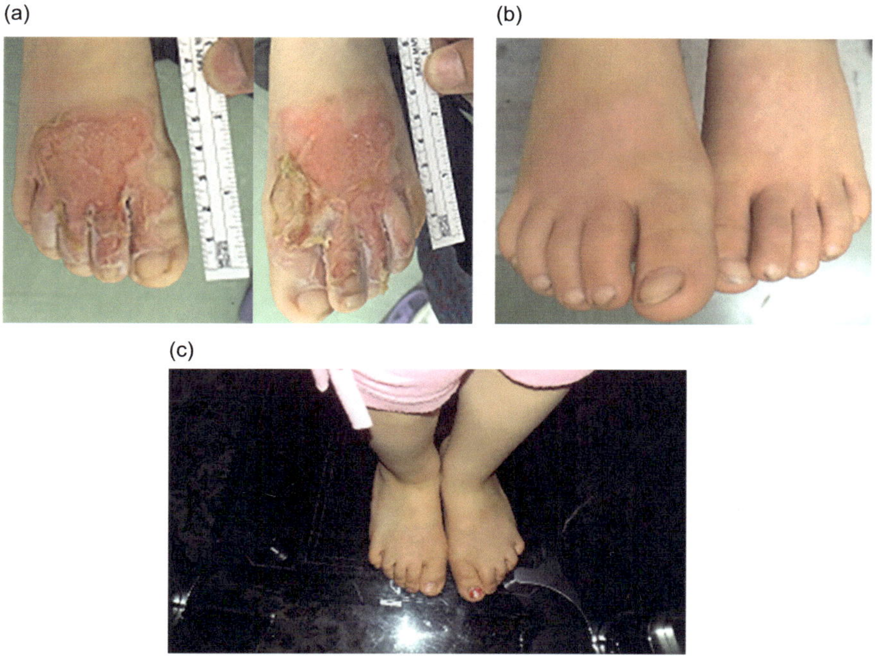

Figure 2.
(a) Grade 2b burn ulcer in a 6-month-old boy present for 2 days before treatment, (b) After 10 sessions of PBM using a 650 nm red laser at 1 J/cm^2. (C) scarless healing observed after 6 m follow up.

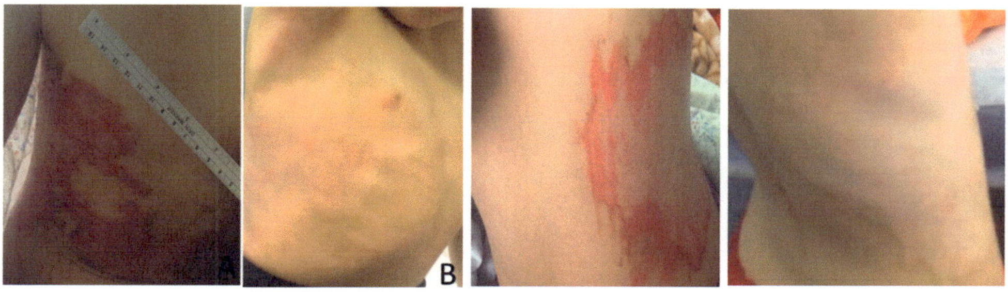

Figure 3.
(a) Grade 2 burn ulcer present for a week prior, (b) After 10 sessions of PBM using a 650 nm red laser, 1 J/cm^2.

2.1 Effect of PBM on scar formation and healing

Scars are commonly formed after trauma, surgery, and especially burns. While some of them heal spontaneously, others may develop into hypertrophic scars and keloids, which are usually hard to treat and have a significant functional and psychological burden for patients. Unfortunately, there is no accepted therapeutic modality to treat these scars completely and permanently. Prevention would be the best treatment. Several randomized controlled trials (RCTs) support the effects of PBM on improving post-burn hypertrophic scars.

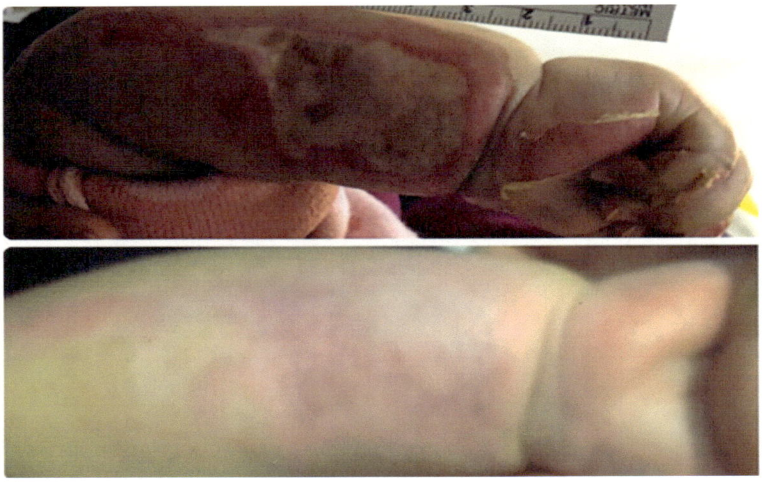

Figure 4.
(a) Grade 3 burn ulcer in a 6-month-old child, 2 weeks pre-treatment, (b) After 12 sessions of PBM using a 650 nm red laser, 1 J/cm^2.

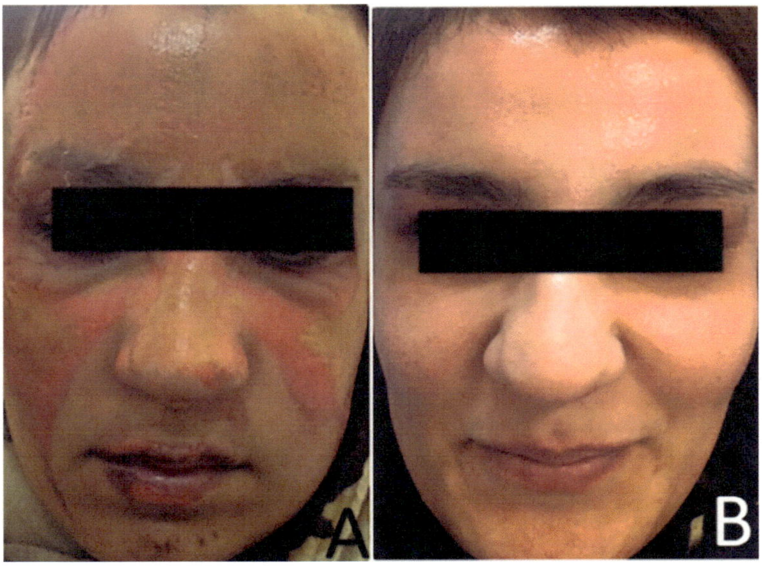

Figure 5.
(a) Grade 2 burn ulcer for 3 days pre-treatment (b) After 10 sessions of PBM using 650 nm red laser, 1 J/cm^2.

To treat hypertrophic scars with PBM, higher doses (10–16 J/cm$_2$) are needed to decrease mitochondrial activity and cell viability. Higher doses also have inhibitory effects on TGF-β. In-vitro studies show that 16 J/cm^2 red and IR laser light increased apoptosis in cultured skin fibroblasts [9, 10] (**Figures 8–10**).

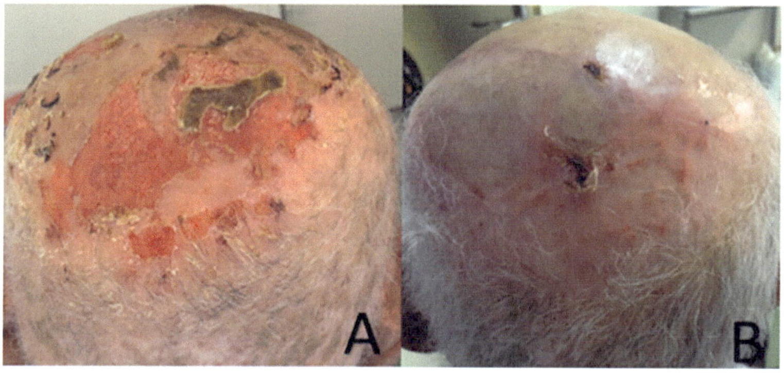

Figure 6.
(a) Grade 3 burn ulcer on the scalp, (b) After 10 sessions of PBM.

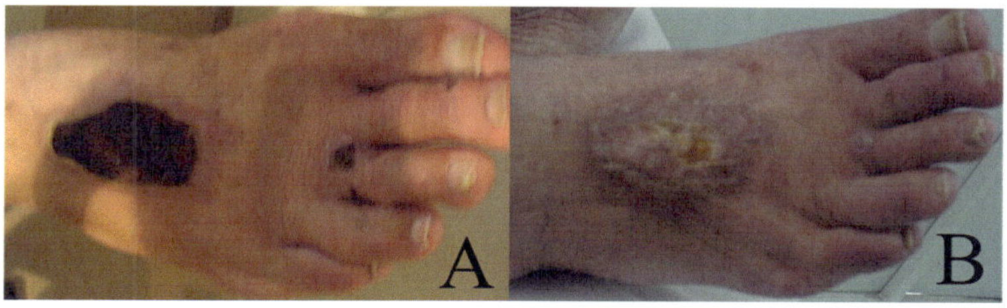

Figure 7.
(a) Grade 3 burn ulcer in a 70-year-old diabetic patient present the past 2 months, (b) after 20 sessions of PBM (3 months), without necrotomy.

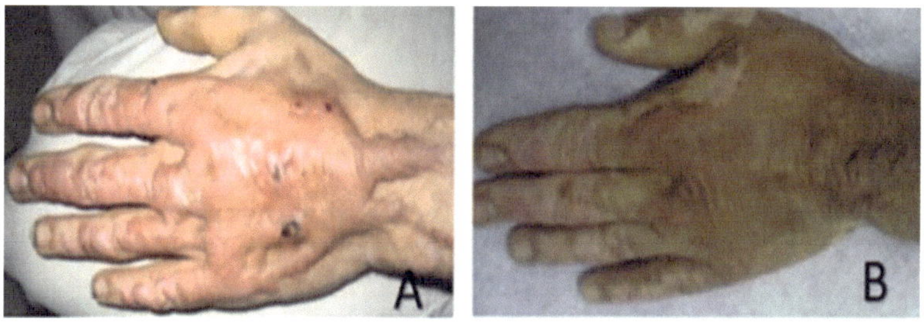

Figure 8.
(a) Post-burn hypertrophic scar in the past 9 months, (b) After 45 sessions of PBM.

2.2 Using PBM in electrical burn ulcers

Electrical burn injuries account for 3%–7% of all hospitalized burns and are the fourth leading cause of traumatic work-related death. Because of the widespread use of electricity, the risk of electrical injuries has increased in developing countries. Electrical burns have greater severity, higher disability and mortality rates, more complicated management, long-term hospitalization, and more costly expenditure, and therefore are perceived as one of the most destructive injuries. They are

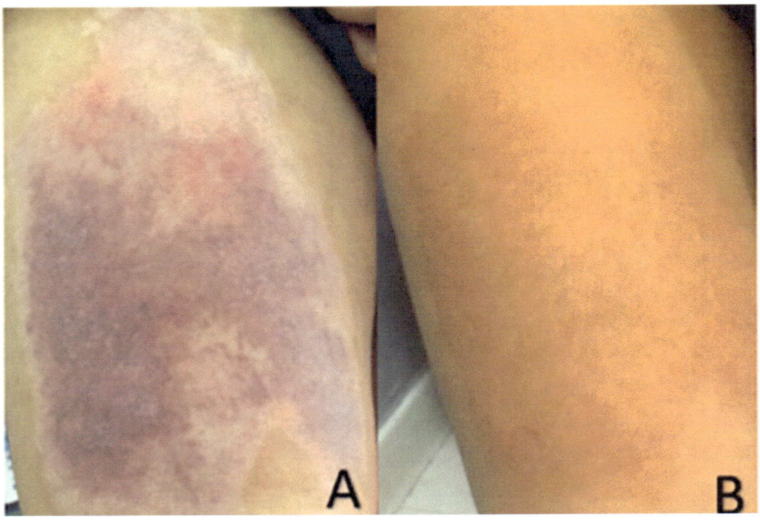

Figure 9.
(a) Post-burn persistent erythema, (b) After 16 sessions of PBM.

considered moderate to severe burn ulcers, and inpatient care is recommended for electrical burns due to high-voltage electric shock to enable systemic monitoring. Electric shocks can cause damage not only to the skin but also to a variety of organs and tissues because of the electrical current flowing through the body. It is difficult to make comparisons between patients as the cause of injury, site of injury, pathway of electrical current, and duration of contact vary widely on a case-by-case basis. Early debridement might be needed to prevent myoglobinemia and kidney damage if muscle tissue has been significantly damaged. The high temperature and direct injury of the current flow to deep tissue might lead to deeper burn depth in electrical burns compared with other burns. Operations, including split-thickness skin grafts (STSGs) and skin flaps might be required in most electrical burn patients. Due to electrical damage to nerves, arteries, and connective tissue, the rate of graft failure and amputation is higher in these patients. Using PBM may be effective in treating dehiscence and graft failure and reducing the rate of repeated surgeries [11] (**Figures 10, 11**).

2.3 Using PBM post-skin graft and flap

Application of PBM is also useful after STSG to accelerate the healing rate and decrease the rate of graft failure, dehiscence, hypertrophic scars, and keloids. In a randomized clinical trial, we selected patients with bilateral, similar grade 3 burn ulcers on both hands and both feet who underwent STSG. One side was selected for laser irradiation and the other side as a control, randomly. The red 655 nm laser was used for irradiation every day for 7 days at a power output of 150 mW, 2 J/cm^2 to the bed of the ulcer, and with infra-red 808 nm light, 200 mW for the margins. The rate of wound dehiscence after STSG was significantly lower in the laser-treated group in comparison with the control group, which received only classic dressing (P = 0.019) [12] (**Figures 12–17**).

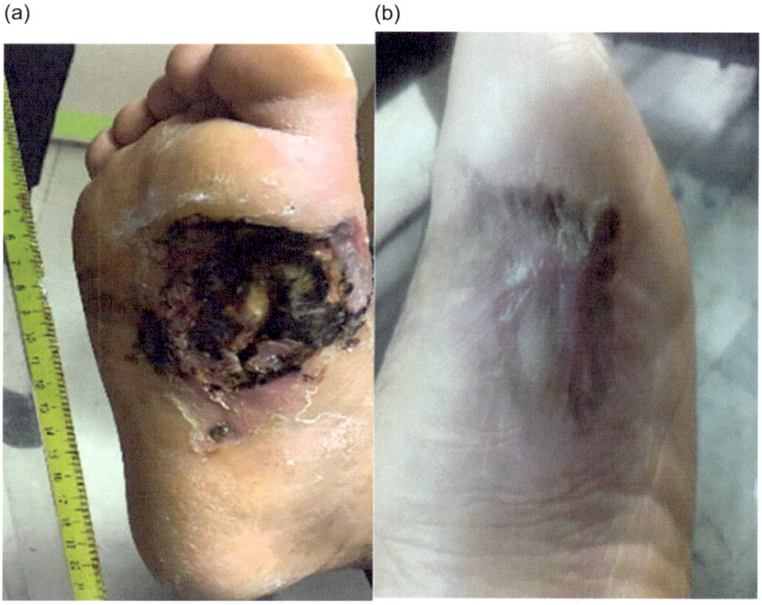

Figure 10.
(a) Electrical burn ulcer in a 40-year-old male for 2 weeks, (b) After 20 sessions of PBM.

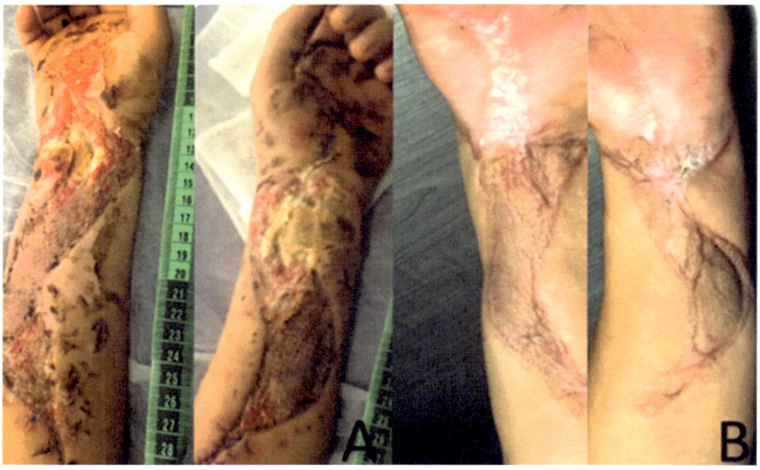

Figure 11.
(a) Skin graft failure after an burn in a 32-year-old man; complete healing occurred after 25 sessions of PBM using red light at 1 J/cm^{2}cm^2 for the open wounds and 6 J/cm^2 IR laser for the margins, administered other day for 12 sessions and then twice per week for 10 sessions.

In our previous study, we compared the prognosis of STSG as the standard treatment for deep burn ulcers with PBM in children. The results showed that local irradiation with a red laser was an effective alternative to surgery and significantly decreased the rate of scar and hypertrophic scar formation, a common complication after burns and surgery ($P < 0.001$). **Figures 1–4** show some of these results. PBM also decreased pain and pruritus, which bother patients during the healing process [6].

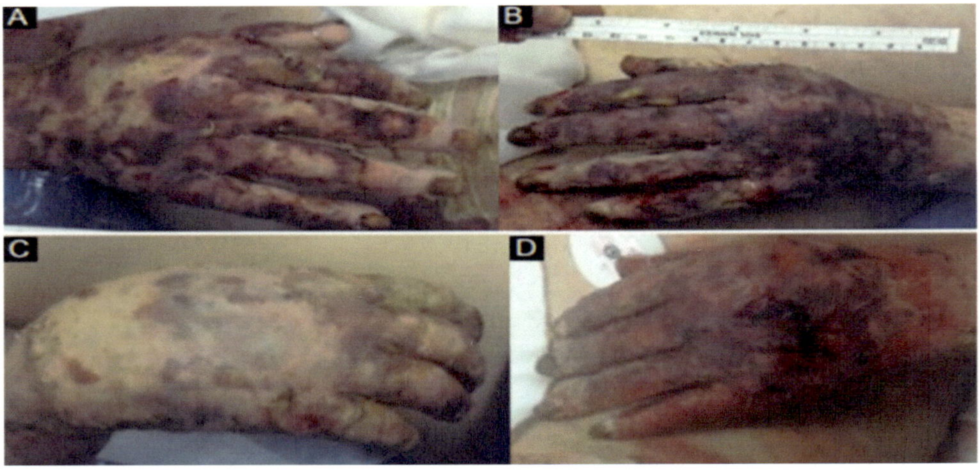

Figure 12.
(a, b) Skin graft for bilateral grade 3 burn ulcers. (c) After 10 sessions of PBM. (d) Control side.

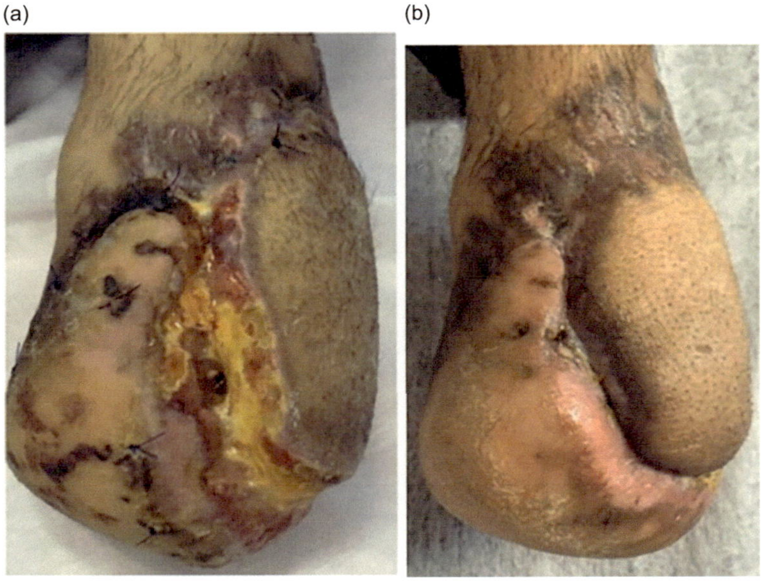

Figure 13.
(a) 24-year-old diabetic patient with grade 3 burn ulcer, dehiscence of ulcer after amputation and flap surgery, candidate for amputation above the ankle, (b) after 15 sessions of PBM.

Managing donor sites after grafting is also very important. Although several modern dressings are available to manage the comfort of the donor site, sometimes patients experience more discomfort at the donor site than at the recipient's burn site itself. PBM accelerates the healing process and may decrease the rate of hypertrophic scar formation. In our previous randomized clinical trial, we selected 18 donor sites in 11 patients with grade 3 burn ulceration. Donor areas were randomly divided into

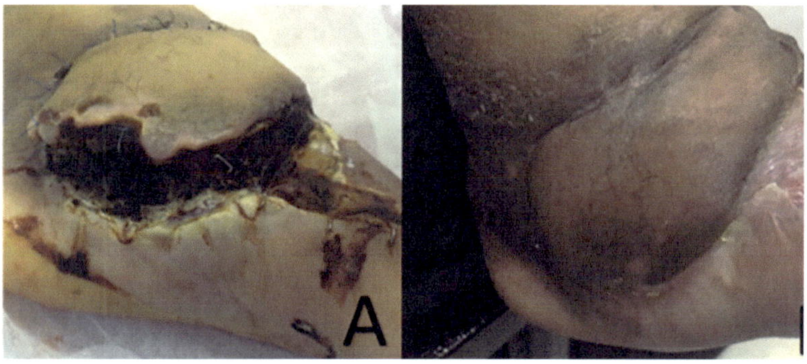

Figure 14.
(a) Wound dehiscence after STSG in a patient with grade 3 burn ulcer, (b) After 10 sessions of PBM.

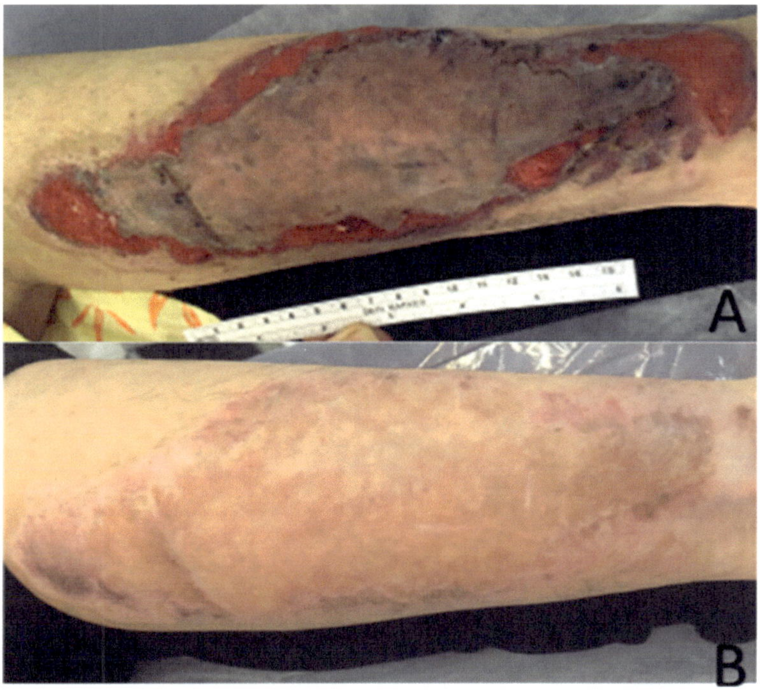

Figure 15.
(a) Dehiscence after skin graft, (b) After 15 sessions of PBM.

two parts: a laser irradiation group and a control group. The laser area was irradiated with a red, 655-nm laser light, 150 mW, 2 J/cm^2, on days 0 (immediately after surgery), 3, 5, and 7. Dressings and other therapeutic care for both sites were the same. The patients and the person who analyzed the results were blinded. The size of the donor site reduced in both groups during the seven-day study period, and this reduction was significantly greater ($P = 0.01$) in the laser group [13] (**Figure 18**).

In another study, we used PBM to treat deep burn ulcers in complicated patients, including diabetics. These patients were candidates for amputation, as STSG, the

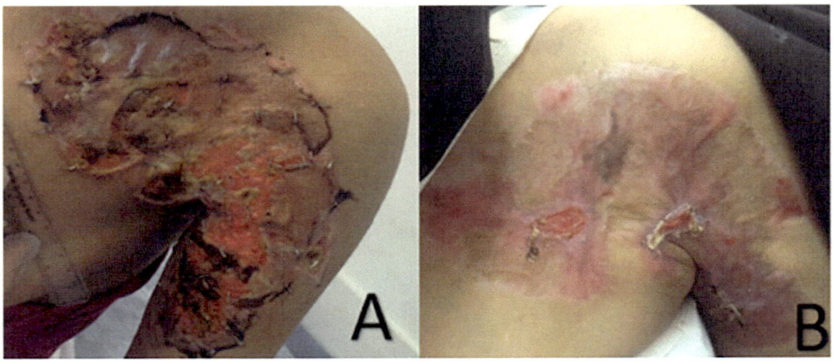

Figure 16.
(a) Grade 3 burn ulcer, graft failure, candidate for second graft surgery. (b) After 12 sessions of PBM.

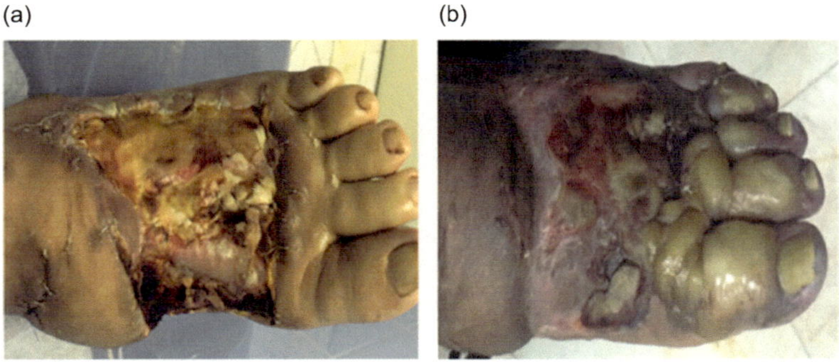

Figure 17.
(a) Graft failure in a burn ulcer in a patient. (b) After 20 of PMB using red and IR lights.

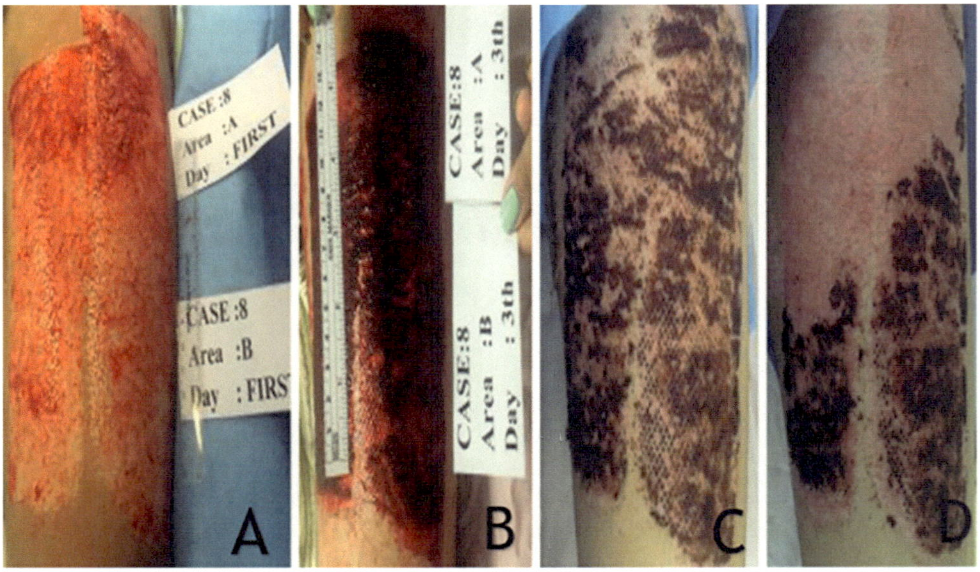

Figure 18.
Pictures of the donor site on days 0, 3, 5, and 7. A is the laser-treated area, and B is the control area.

standard treatment for deep burn ulcers, was not suitable for them. After 15–30 sessions of PBM using a 650 nm red laser at 1 J/cm^2 for the bed of the ulcer and an 810 nm IR laser at 4 J/cm^2 for the margins, enough granulation tissue covered the bed of the ulcer, enabling the surgeon to perform STSG. To decrease the chance of graft failure, which is a common complication in diabetic patients, PBM using IR at 4 J/cm^2 was continued until complete healing [14] (**Figures 19–24**).

2.4 PBM for treating post-burn depigmentation

Grades 2 and 3 burn injuries may heal with changes in pigmentation. Occasionally, depigmentation may become permanent, especially in the hands, wrists, and fingers, which may become a psychological burden for patients. Although many unknown causes are responsible for post-burn depigmentation, most scholars believe that melanocyte destruction or loss from the basal layers plays a major role. Scar formation in the skin may also be an obstacle to melanocyte migration from adjacent intact areas. There are two sources for re-pigmentation: the first from melanocyte stem cells located in the hair follicles and the second from

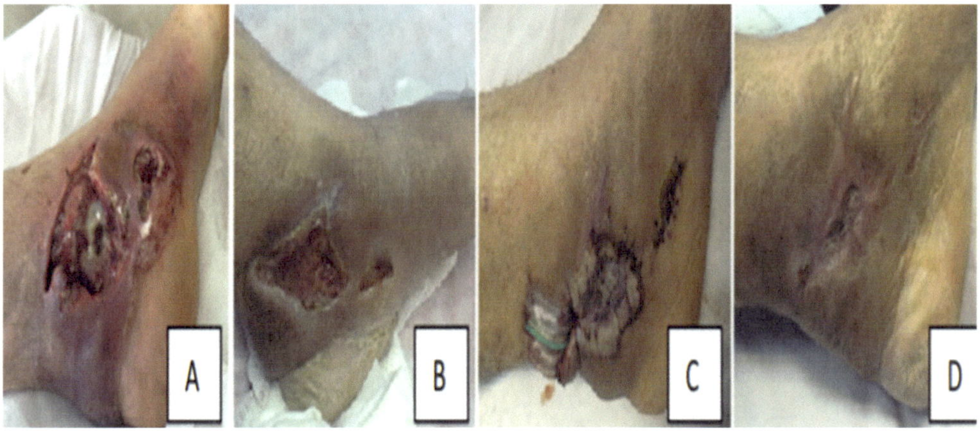

Figure 19.
(a) Grade 3 burn ulcer in a 47-year-old diabetic man 6 months ago pre-treatment, (b) granulation tissue coverage after 10 sessions of PBM, (c) STSG, (d) after 3 months follow up.

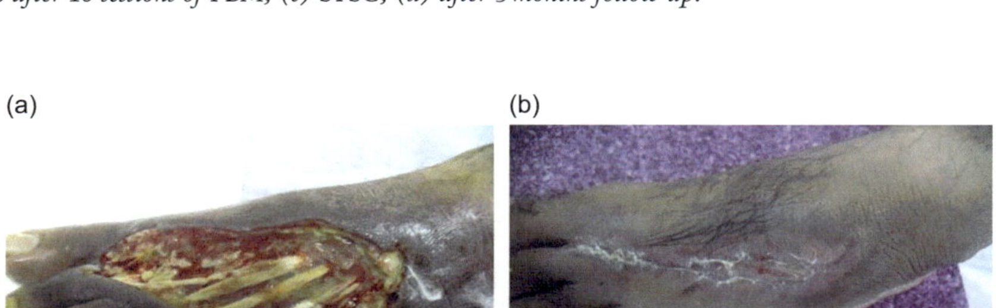

Figure 20.
(a) Deep burn ulcer in a 40-year-old diabetic, 3 months pre-treatment. (b) After 39 sessions of PBM using red and IR light.

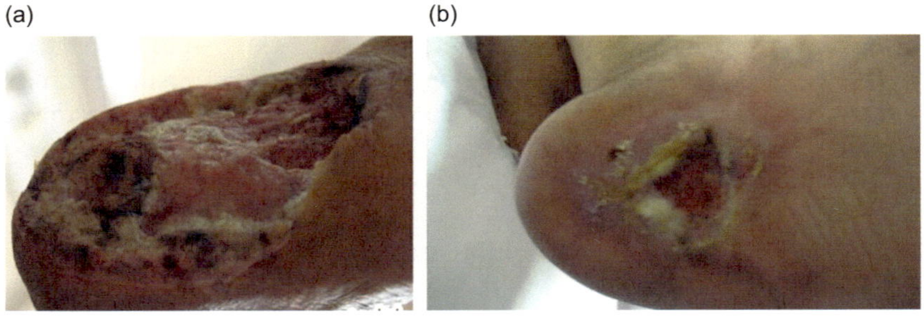

Figure 21.
(a) Deep burn ulcer in a 45-year-old diabetic patient for 2 months. (b) After 120 sessions of PBM using red and IR light.

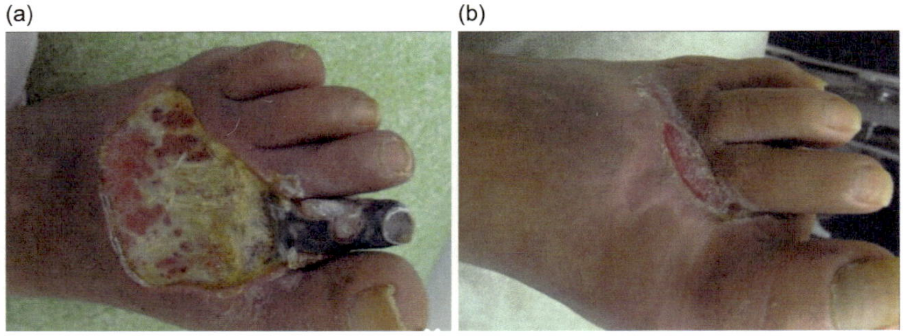

Figure 22.
(a) Deep burn ulcer in a diabetic patient for 2 years, (b) After 30 sessions of PBM using red and IR light.

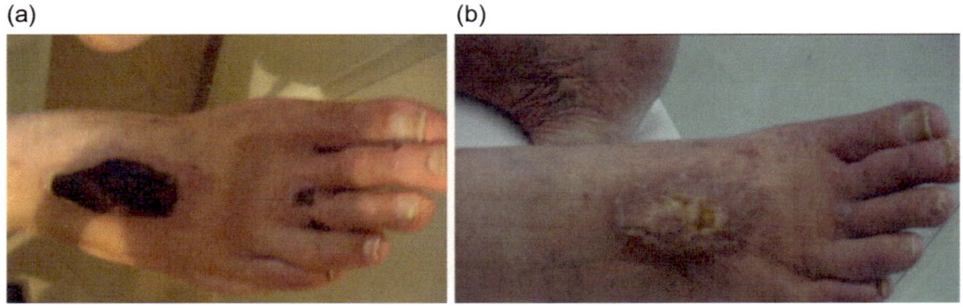

Figure 23.
(a) Necrotic burn ulcer in a diabetic patient for 2 months. (b) After 19 sessions of PBM, without necrotomy debridement.

adjacent intact epidermis. Skin grafts and cellular grafts (melanocyte transplantation) are the main surgical treatment modalities. PBM may also induce the re-pigmentation process in vitiligo. He–Ne red light laser has been reported to induce the activation and proliferation of melanocyte precursors. Blue light also activates melanocytes through the opsin-3 (OPS3) signaling pathway [15, 16]. We

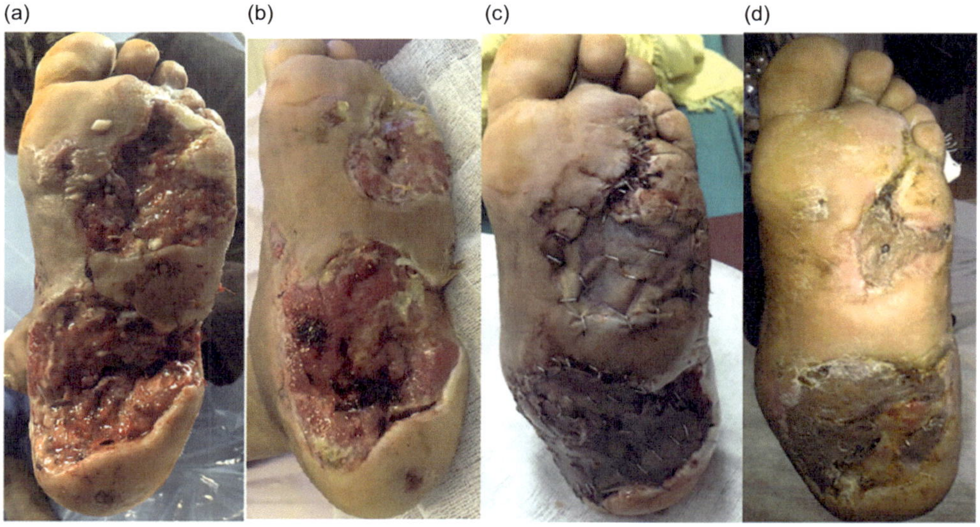

Figure 24.
(a) Deep burn ulcer in a patient for 3 months, (b) After 10 sessions of PBM using red and IR, (c) STSG and IR illumination, (d) after 15 sessions of PBM.

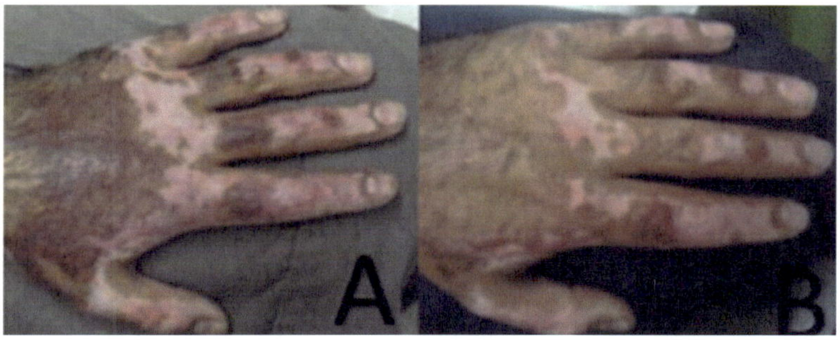

Figure 25.
Post-burn depigmentation one month before treatment. After 24 sessions of PBM using an 810 nm laser at 6 J/cm^2 (12 sessions, 3 times per week, followed by 10 sessions, 2 times per week).

used an IR 810 nm laser, 6 J/cm^2 for post-burn depigmentation, which is beneficial, especially if treatment is started early (**Figure 25**).

3. How to treat burn ulcers using PBM

The most common wavelengths used in wound healing are red and near-infrared (NIR). Red light has the greatest stimulatory effect on wound healing; however, due to higher absorption by the vascular skin network, it has less penetration depth – less than 10 mm. Therefore, red light is mainly applied to the exposed bed of the ulcer. NIR penetrates deeper into the tissue and is applied to the wound's margins to increase fibroblast and epithelial cell proliferation and enhance perfusion [17].

Red light, in the 620–700 nanometer (nm) range, with common effective wavelengths including 630 nm and 660 nm, and a dose of 1–2 J/cm^2 is usually used to illuminate the bed of the ulcer to stimulate the wound healing process.

NIR 810–850 nm, 4–6 J/cm^2, is recommended for the margins to stimulate cellular migration, re-epithelialization, and increase perfusion.

It is recommended to do 2–3 sessions of treatment per week for up to 10–12 sessions, and then 1–2 sessions per week until complete recovery.

Light can be illuminated from a 1–2 cm distance to avoid contamination (**Figure 26**), or through a sterile, transparent cover for the direct contact method (**Figure 27**).

Important point: Using IR light over the growth plates is contraindicated in children.

To ensure accurate light dosing and to avoid overdosing, it is recommended that irradiation points be spaced approximately 1 cm apart, with no overlaps between adjacent points (**Figure 28**).

4. Contraindications of PBM

There are several contraindications for PBM in the literature. Some of them are, however, quite useless; their correctness has never been demonstrated. These result in a few mistakes, and physicians sometimes discourage patient use, although the application of the therapeutic laser would be beneficial. Thus, the contraindications can be divided into the following three principal groups: (1) justified, (2) doubtful under certain conditions, and (3) erroneous. However, further studies might change the situation.

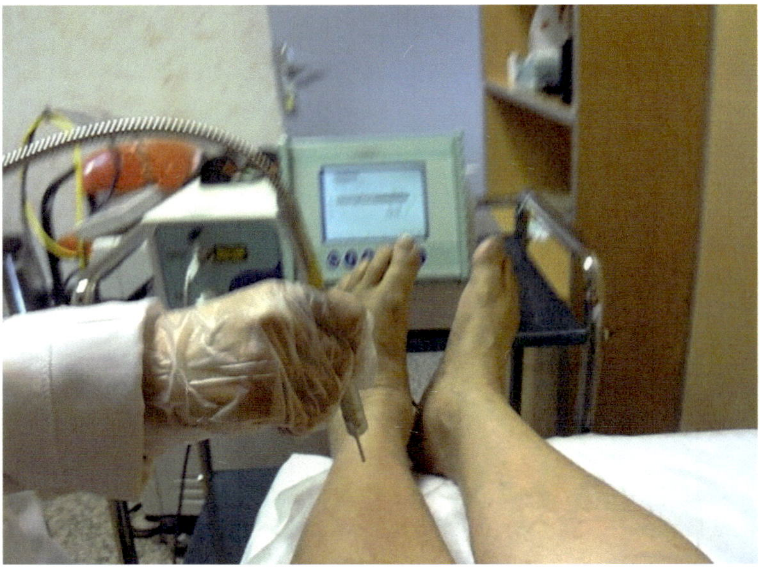

Figure 26.
Non-direct light illumination.

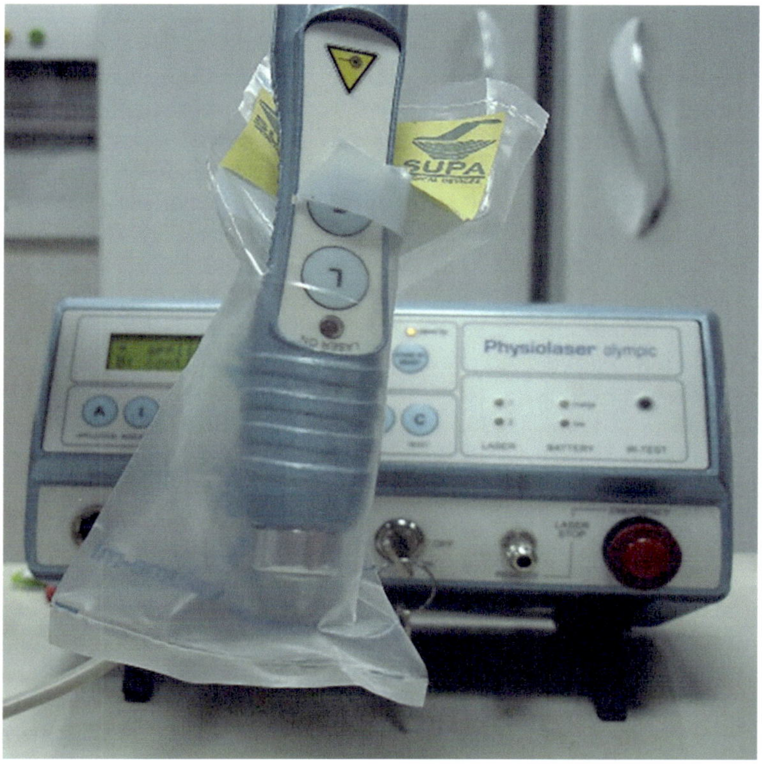

Figure 27.
Direct light illumination through a transparent, sterile cover.

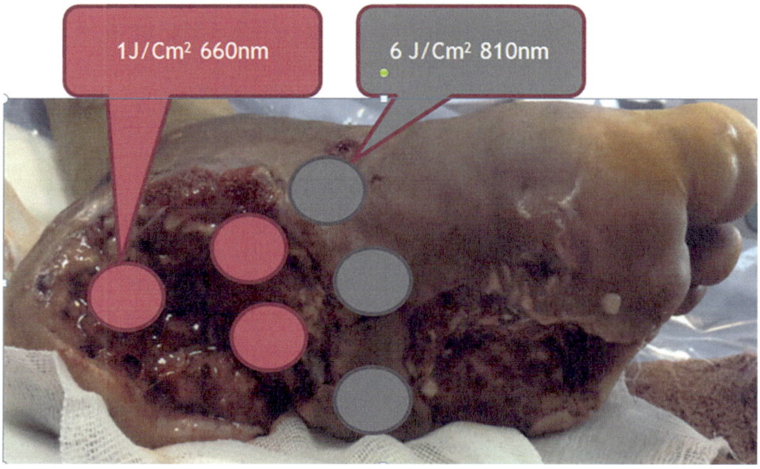

Figure 28.
How to illuminate light on the wound.

4.1 Using PBM in malignancies

There were always doubts regarding the use of PBM over a tumor. In a systematic review conducted in 2020, some studies reported an increase in cell proliferation, while others showed a decrease. Theoretically, the bio-stimulating effect is induced through activation of the respiratory chain enzymes. The higher the ATP utilization in tissues, the more rapid the ADP production, and thus the more rapid the aerobic phosphorylation. As PBM increases the concentrations of ATP, ADP, and adenosine monophosphate in the cell, it induces an accelerated replication of mitochondrial DNA5,6 and the G0–S phase. PBM also enhances the consumption of oxygen and glucose and accelerates metabolism locally. Since this condition could also be induced at a site not directly exposed to the laser beam, it was assumed that the bio-stimulating effect of surface irradiation could also be mediated by humoral factors. Thus, PBM was assumed to be contraindicated in all patients with malignancies [18]. However, experiments on the effect of PBM on cultured cells are not representative of the *in vivo* condition. *In vivo* studies on mice show that laser light might be able to reduce tumor progression, suggesting that PBM might be a safe procedure in multi-modal anticancer protocols in humans. Some studies suggest that photobiomodulation therapy induces apoptosis and cell death in malignant neoplastic cells in a dose-dependent manner, lacking the potential to activate residual malignant cells. Due to the lack of standardization of laser irradiation protocols and ideal parameters for this purpose, PBM should be used with caution in cancer patients until more studies are performed [19]. Every case must be considered individually, but as a rule, using PBM is not recommended for patients with known or suspected neoplasia or tumors and their margins. However, it might be acceptable if the tumor has been removed and the margins are clear. Current data shows it is acceptable to use PBM at sites distant from the tumor. Several review articles and RCTs support the safety and efficacy of PBM in the prevention and treatment of oral mucositis in patients undergoing radiotherapy and chemotherapy for head and neck cancer, leukemia, lymphoma, and acute lymphoblastic leukemia. When in doubt, distal or systemic effects on regional lymph nodes or blood irradiation might be useful [20].

4.2 Pregnancy

In literature, using a laser over the abdominal area with high doses is reported as a contraindication. However, there is no scientific evidence to support the risk of irradiation of areas distant from the gravid uterus. Available evidence, limited to low evidence-level case reports and series, indicates that cutaneous laser treatment during pregnancy is safe for both the fetus and the mother. It is suggested that, according to laser physics and optics, there should theoretically be no risk of fetal laser exposure from commonly used cutaneous lasers [21].

4.3 Head and neck area

PBM might decrease thyroglobulin mRNA and stimulate TSH. With respect to a possible bio stimulating effect, PBM should be applied with maximum caution in the neck region and the thyroid region should be avoided to prevent possibly inducing hyperthyroidism, although PBM is used safely for treating hypothyroidism [22]. Some researchers have indicated the periocular area and exposure of the retina as contraindications for laser treatment, but it's safe with proper eye coverage [23].

4.4 Pacemakers

Pacemakers were previously considered a contraindication, but as they are metallic instruments, PBM has no effect on them [24].

5. Laser safety: Risks and hazards

Now a days, besides hospitals and operating rooms, laser technology is available in office practices, clinics, and private enterprises, so the responsibility for laser safety falls on individual users as well. The goal is to establish a laser-safe environment for users and patients. Proper safety requires knowledge of standards, identification of hazards and risks, implementation of appropriate control measures, and consistent program audits to demonstrate quality assurance. Laser users should have knowledge of exposure limits, maximum permissible exposure, ocular hazards, classification, etc.

The potential PBM hazards are mostly ocular, especially for laser devices. Ocular injury levels depend on the laser-tissue interaction, power and energy density, and clinical application technique. Long-wavelength lasers like CO2 and Er:YAG are absorbed by the water in the tissue, so they can be absorbed at the tear layer covering the cornea. This is not permanent but might be painful and temporarily disabling. Short-wavelength near-infrared and visible ranges can transmit through all anterior structures of the eye, be absorbed by the hemoglobin in the retina, and cause permanent damage to central vision.

In most cases, PBM devices are class 3B or LED-based, but sometimes defocused class IV lasers might also be used. Most PBM devices emit divergent beams (not focused or collimated), so the ocular risk diminishes over distance. Laser beams must not be aimed into the eyes, and everyone present should wear appropriate safety spectacles. Safety precautions, including eye protection, reflection, flammability, and administrative control measures, are determined by the classification of lasers.

Photothermal wavelength of 10,600 (Carbon dioxide) can create enough heat to cause a flammability hazard, so alcohol-containing solutions, sources of oxygen, flammable gases, and dry materials must be removed from the target zone [23].

6. Conclusion(s)

Based on the literature review and more than two decades of the author's clinical experience, PBM can be effectively used to accelerate the healing process and reduce complications, including scars and hypertrophic scars, in burn ulcers. PBM is a painless, safe, and cost-benefit therapeutic modality compared to other conventional treatments.

Acknowledgments

The authors would like to express their sincere gratitude to all colleagues and hospital staff whose dedication and support contributed to the care and treatment of the patients, and special thanks to the patients who participated in the studies and generously granted permission for the publication of their clinical photographs.

Conflict of Interest

The authors declare no conflict of interest.

Author details

Nooshafarin Kazemikhoo[1*] and Chow A.M. Roberta[2]

1 Hunter NewEngland Health, Newcastle, Australia

2 Brain and Mind Center, University of Sydney & Quantum Pain Management, Sydney, Australia

*Address all correspondence to: nooshafarin.kazemikhoo@health.nsw.gov.au; nooshakazemi@gmail.com

References

[1] Priyadarski A, Gaurav K, Gupta A. Dual-NIR wavelength (pulsed 810 nm and superpulsed 904 nm lasers) photobiomodulation therapy synergistically augments full-thickness burn wound healing: A non-invasive approach. Journal of Photochemistry and Photobiology. 2023;**246**:1276. DOI: 10.1016/j.jphotobiol.2023.112761

[2] Woodruff LD, Bounkeo JM, Brannon WM, Dawes KS, Barham CD, Waddell DL, et al. The efficacy of laser therapy in wound repair: A meta-analysis of the literature. Photomedicine and Laser Surgery 2004;**22**:241–247

[3] Kaviani A, Djavid GE, Ataie-Fashtami L, Fateh M, Ghodsi M, Salami M, et al. A randomized clinical trial on the effect of low-level laser therapy on chronic diabetic foot wound healing: A preliminary report. Photomedicine and Laser Surgery 2011;**29**:109–114

[4] Tang E, Khan I, Andreana S, Arany P. Laser-activated transforming growth factor-β1 induces human β-defensin 2: Implications for laser therapies for periodontitis and peri-implantitis. Journal of Periodontal Research. 2017;**52**(3):360–367

[5] Khoo NK, Shokrgozar MA, Kashani IR, Amanzadeh A, Mostafavi E, Sanati H, et al. In vitro therapeutic effects of a low-level laser at mRNA level on the release of skin growth factors from fibroblasts in diabetic mice. Avicenna Journal of Medical Biotechnology 2014;**6**:113–118

[6] Kazemikhoo N, et al. Effects of photobiomodulation and split-thickness skin grafting in the prognosis of wound healing in children with deep burn ulcers. Photobiomodulation, Photomedicine, and Laser Surgery 2022;**40**:148–154

[7] Rahmannia M, Amini A, Chien S, Bayat M. Impact of photobiomodulation on macrophages and their polarization during diabetic wound healing: A systematic review. Lasers in Medical Science. 2022;**37**(7):2805–2815

[8] Khan I, Rahman SU, Tang E, Engel K, Hall B, Kulkarni AB, Arany PR. Accelerated burn wound healing with photobiomodulation therapy involves activation of endogenous latent TGF-β1. Scientific Reports. 2021;**11**(1):13371

[9] Kim YH, Kim HK, Choi JW, Kim YC. Photobiomodulation therapy with an 830-nm light-emitting diode for the prevention of thyroidectomy scars: A randomized, double-blind, sham device-controlled clinical trial. Lasers in Medical Science. 2022;**37**(9):3583–3590

[10] Alsharnoubi J, Mohamed O, Fawzy M. Photobiomodulation effect on children's scars. Lasers in Medical Science. 2018;**33**(3):497–501

[11] Ocon CA, Dos Santos SA, Caires JR, de Oliveira MF, Serra AJ, Leal-Junior EC, de Carvalho PD. Effects and parameters of the photobiomodulation in experimental models of third-degree burn: Systematic review. Lasers in Medical Science. 2019;**34**(3):637–648

[12] Kazemikhoo N, Vaghardoost R, Dahmardehei M, Mokmeli S, Momeni M, Nilforoushzadeh MA, Ansari F, Razagi MR, Razagi Z, Amirkhani MA, Masjedi MR.

Evaluation of the effects of low level laser therapy on the healing process after skin graft surgery in burned patients (a randomized clinical trial). Journal of Lasers in Medical Sciences. 2018;**9**(2):139

[13] Vaghardoost R, Momeni M, Kazemikhoo N, Mokmeli S, Dahmardehei M, Ansari F, Nilforoushzadeh MA, Joo PS, Abadi SM, Gharagheshlagh SN, Sassani S. Effect of lowlevel laser therapy on the healing process of donor site in patients with grade 3 burn ulcer after skin graft surgery (a randomised clinical trial). Lasers in Medical Science. 2018;**33**(3):603–607. DOI: 10.1007/s10103-017-2430-4

[14] Dahmardehei M, Kazemikhoo N, Vaghardoost R, Mokmeli S, Momeni M, Nilforoushzadeh MA, Ansari F, Amirkhani A. Effects of low level laser therapy on the prognosis of split-thickness skin graft in type 3 burn of diabetic patients: A case series. Lasers in Medical Science. 2016;**31**(3):497–502

[15] de Araújo Pereira Venceslau SC, Ferreira JL, Barros RM, de Morais RM, Dos Santos HH, de Oliveira VM, de Andrade PR. Effects of photobiomodulation on re-epithelialization of burn wound: Protocol for a randomized controlled trial. Trials. 2022;**23**(1):573

[16] Orlandi C, Purpura V, Melandri D. Blue led light in burns: A new treatment's modality. Journal of Clinical and Investigative Dermatology. 2021;**9**(5)

[17] Yadav A, Gupta A. Noninvasive red and near-infrared wavelength-induced photobiomodulation: Promoting impaired cutaneous wound healing. Photodermatology, Photoimmunology & Photomedicine. 2017;**33**(1):4–13

[18] Bensadoun RJ, Epstein JB, Nair RG, Barasch A, Raber-Durlacher JE, Migliorati C, Genot-Klastersky MT, Treister N, Arany P, Lodewijckx J, Robijns J. Safety and efficacy of photobiomodulation therapy in oncology: A systematic review. Cancer Medicine. 2020;**9**(22):8279–8300

[19] Hamblin MR, Nelson ST, Strahan JR. Photobiomodulation and cancer: What is the truth? Photomedicine and Laser Surgery. 2018;**36**(5):241–245

[20] Courtois E, Bouleftour W, Guy JB, Louati S, Bensadoun RJ, Rodriguez-Lafrasse C, Magné N. Mechanisms of PhotoBioModulation (PBM) focused on oral mucositis prevention and treatment: A scoping review. BMC Oral Health. 2021;**21**(1):220

[21] Traverzim MA, Sobral AP, Fernandes KP, de Fátima Teixeira Silva D, Pavani C, Mesquita-Ferrari RA, Horliana AC, Gomes AO, Bussadori SK, Motta LJ. The effect of photobiomodulation on analgesia during childbirth: A controlled and randomized clinical trial. Photobiomodulation, Photomedicine, and Laser Surgery. 2021;**39**(4):265–271

[22] Berisha-Muharremi V, Tahirbegolli B, Phypers R, Hanna R. Efficacy of combined photobiomodulation therapy with supplements versus supplements alone in restoring thyroid gland homeostasis in Hashimoto thyroiditis: A clinical feasibility parallel trial with 6-months follow-up. Journal of Personalized Medicine. 2023;**13**(8):1274

[23] Mota LR, Duarte ID, Galache TR, Pretti KM, Neto OC, Motta LJ, Horliana AC, Silva DD, Pavani C. Photobiomodulation reduces periocular

wrinkle volume by 30%: A randomized controlled trial. Photobiomodulation, Photomedicine, and Laser Surgery. 2023;**41**(2):48–56

[24] Parker S, Cronshaw M. Laser safety in dental practice in the United Kingdom: Laser safety in dental practice in the United Kingdom. British Dental Journal. 2025;**238**(11):879–888

Section 5

Long-Term Outcomes and Sequelae

Chapter 9

Comprehensive Approaches to Burn Scar Management

Chandler Hinson, Kimberly A. Donnellan, Andrew C. Bright and Kevin Slaughter

Abstract

This chapter provides a comprehensive, structured overview of contemporary burn scar prevention and management, integrating pathophysiology, clinical classification, and treatment strategies across the continuum of care. It begins with an introduction to the global burden of burn injury and the long-term functional, aesthetic, and psychosocial consequences of scarring. The chapter then outlines key biological mechanisms, including inflammatory signaling, fibroblast activation, myofibroblast persistence, and dysregulated collagen remodeling, which underpin hypertrophic scars, keloids, and contractures. Subsequent sections classify burn scars and detail conservative management, emphasizing pressure therapy, silicone application, massage, and early rehabilitation to mitigate fibrosis and preserve mobility. Advanced therapies, including laser modalities, intralesional pharmacotherapy, and surgical reconstruction, are reviewed within evidence-based algorithms tailored to scar maturity and functional impairment. The chapter further explores emerging regenerative approaches, such as fat grafting, stem cell–based therapies, biomaterials, and photobiomodulation, highlighting their potential to restore tissue architecture and improve outcomes. A dedicated section underscores the critical role of multidisciplinary care, integrating surgical, rehabilitative, and psychosocial expertise to optimize recovery. Finally, the chapter addresses long-term surveillance, patient education, and future directions in antifibrotic and regenerative science. Collectively, this framework supports a holistic, patient-centered approach to improving function, appearance, and quality of life for burn survivors worldwide. By aligning early prevention with timely intervention, clinicians can reduce disability, limit recurrence, and enhance durable outcomes across diverse care settings. Emphasis on individualized treatment planning and adherence further strengthens long-term success in burn scar management. Continued innovation and global collaboration will be essential to advance equitable access worldwide.

Keywords: hypertrophic scar, contracture, scar management, wound healing, compression therapy, laser therapy, corticosteroids, surgical scar revision, regenerative medicine

1. Introduction

Burn injuries remain among the most devastating forms of trauma, affecting more than 11 million people globally each year [1]. While the incidence of severe burns in high-income countries has declined to approximately 2–5 cases per 100,000 population due to improved safety standards and acute care systems, the burden remains disproportionately high in low- and middle-income countries (LMIC), where rates exceed 20–30 cases per 100,000 and account for over 90% of burn-related mortality [2, 3]. Consequently, burns rank among the leading causes of disability-adjusted life years lost in LMIC settings [4]. While advances in acute burn care have dramatically improved survival rates, the sequelae of scarring continue to impose a profound burden on survivors – functionally, esthetically, and psychosocially. The resulting scars can lead to disfigurement, restricted mobility, chronic pain, pruritus, and social stigmatization, all of which significantly impair quality of life long after the initial injury.

The process of burn wound healing is inherently complex, involving the interplay of inflammation, angiogenesis, fibroblast proliferation, and extracellular matrix (ECM) remodeling. When dysregulated, this cascade results in excessive collagen deposition, aberrant fibroblast activity, and persistent myofibroblast contraction – hallmarks of hypertrophic scarring and contracture formation. Understanding these underlying mechanisms is critical for tailoring interventions that not only prevent pathological scar formation but also promote optimal functional and aesthetic recovery.

Scar management in burns encompasses a continuum of care that begins in the acute phase of injury and extends through long-term rehabilitation. Effective management requires a multidisciplinary approach, integrating surgical expertise, rehabilitative therapy, psychosocial support, and patient education. Early intervention – through techniques such as pressure garments, silicone application, and guided physical/occupational therapy – plays a pivotal role in mitigating excessive fibrosis. For established scars, a broad range of procedural and surgical options – including laser resurfacing, intralesional pharmacotherapy, and reconstructive techniques – offers avenues for improving pliability, appearance, and function.

Recent years have witnessed rapid expansion in regenerative and technological innovations that aim to restore scarred skin to a more normal phenotype. Fat grafting, stem cell therapy, biomaterial scaffolds, and photobiomodulation (PBM) represent the forefront of a new paradigm in scar modulation, focusing on regeneration rather than mere revision. These approaches complement established modalities and promise to redefine what is achievable in postburn reconstruction.

Ultimately, comprehensive scar management is not a singular intervention but a dynamic and iterative process that adapts to each patient's evolving needs. It requires the coordination of surgeons, physiotherapists, occupational therapists, psychologists, and nursing specialists, all working in concert to optimize outcomes. This chapter provides a detailed, evidence-based overview of the biological mechanisms, preventive strategies, and therapeutic modalities currently shaping the landscape of burn scar management, highlighting both established principles and emerging innovations that are driving the field toward functional and aesthetic restoration.

2. Pathophysiology of burn scar formation

Burn wound healing is a dynamic, multifactorial process that unfolds in overlapping phases of inflammation, proliferation, and remodeling. While the ultimate goal of this cascade is tissue repair and barrier restoration, the process often leads to excessive fibrosis and scar formation when dysregulated. Understanding the molecular and cellular mechanisms underlying this aberrant healing response is essential for the prevention and treatment of hypertrophic scars, keloids, and contractures that frequently follow burn injuries.

2.1 Inflammatory phase and cytokine dysregulation

The inflammatory phase begins immediately after injury with hemostasis and the recruitment of neutrophils and macrophages. These immune cells release a complex network of cytokines, including interleukin-1β (IL-1β), tumor necrosis factor-α (TNF-α), and transforming growth factor-β (TGF-β), which orchestrate cellular migration and matrix deposition [5, 6]. In burn wounds, the depth and extent of tissue necrosis produce prolonged inflammation, maintaining high local concentrations of profibrotic mediators. Persistent macrophage activation and delayed resolution of inflammation amplify fibroblast recruitment and myofibroblast differentiation, establishing a profibrotic milieu that favors abnormal scarring [7].

2.2 Fibroblast activation and myofibroblast differentiation

Fibroblasts are central to scar formation, serving as the primary source of ECM proteins such as collagen types I and III. Under the influence of TGF-β1, connective tissue growth factor (CTGF), and mechanical stress, these fibroblasts differentiate into myofibroblasts, characterized by α-smooth muscle actin (α-SMA) expression and contractile activity [8, 9]. Myofibroblasts play a crucial role in wound contraction; however, in burn wounds, their persistence beyond the normal healing window results in excessive contractile force, collagen cross-linking, and increased tissue stiffness. The failure of apoptosis or reversion to quiescent fibroblasts sustains this cycle, leading to hypertrophic scarring and contracture development [10].

2.3 Collagen deposition and ECM remodeling

In normal wound healing, collagen synthesis and degradation remain in balance through the coordinated action of matrix metalloproteinases (MMPs) and their tissue inhibitors (TIMPs) [11]. Burn scars, however, exhibit excessive deposition of disorganized collagen bundles, a reduced type III to type I collagen ratio, and impaired MMP activity [12, 13]. The dense, parallel collagen architecture seen in hypertrophic scars contrasts with the basket-weave pattern of normal dermis, resulting in decreased elasticity and increased tensile strength [14]. Prolonged fibroblast activity, combined with altered ECM remodeling, perpetuates the cycle of stiffness and mechanical tension that further stimulates fibroblast proliferation – a positive feedback loop that reinforces fibrosis.

2.4 Angiogenesis, hypoxia, and mechanical forces

Burn wounds often exist in a state of relative hypoxia, triggering the expression of hypoxia-inducible factor-1α (HIF-1α) and downstream angiogenic mediators such as vascular endothelial growth factor (VEGF) [15]. While these factors are initially beneficial for revascularization, chronic hypoxia and unstable neovascularization can promote fibrosis through continued TGF-β signaling [16]. In addition, mechanical tension – resulting from underlying muscle movement, wound contraction, and joint motion – acts as a potent stimulus for myofibroblast persistence [17]. This mechanotransduction reinforces the fibrotic phenotype and explains the predilection of hypertrophic scars for high-tension regions such as the neck, shoulders, and joints.

2.5 Neurogenic and immunologic modulation

Emerging research highlights the role of neurogenic inflammation and immune dysregulation in burn scar pathogenesis. Sensory nerve fibers release neuropeptides such as substance P and calcitonin gene–related peptide (CGRP), which promote vasodilation, fibroblast proliferation, and inflammatory cytokine release [18, 19]. In parallel, an imbalance between Th1 and Th2 immune responses – favoring Th2-dominant, profibrotic signaling – contributes to sustained collagen synthesis and impaired remodeling [20]. These neuroimmunologic interactions help explain symptoms such as pruritus and dysesthesia commonly associated with burn scars.

3. Classification of burn scars

The clinical manifestations of burn scarring represent a continuum of aberrant wound-healing responses that vary in morphology, biological activity, and functional consequences. Accurate classification of burn scars is critical not only for diagnosis and prognostication but also for guiding therapeutic decision-making and evaluating treatment outcomes. While burn scars may be broadly categorized by their histopathologic and clinical features, three principal types are recognized and utilized: hypertrophic scars, keloids, and contractures. These entities share overlapping molecular mechanisms but differ in their extent, duration, and tissue behavior.

3.1 Hypertrophic scars

Hypertrophic scars are the most common form of pathologic scarring following deep dermal or full-thickness burns. They are characterized by raised, erythematous, and firm lesions that remain confined within the original wound boundaries (see **Figure 1**). Histologically, they exhibit dense collagen deposition arranged in parallel or whorled bundles, abundant myofibroblasts, and increased vascularity – findings consistent with ongoing remodeling and mechanical tension within the scar bed [21, 22].

Hypertrophic scars typically develop within weeks of wound closure and reach their peak thickness within 3–6 months. Unlike keloids, they often regress spontaneously over 12–24 months as fibroblast activity diminishes and collagen remodeling progresses. The likelihood of hypertrophic scar formation correlates with prolonged wound healing (>3 weeks), infection, and high-tension anatomic sites such as the shoulders, neck, and joints [12, 23]. These scars may cause significant pruritus, pain, and stiffness, particularly when overlying joints, leading to functional impairment.

3.2 Keloids

Keloids represent an exaggerated fibroproliferative response in which scar tissue extends beyond the margins of the original wound and fails to regress over time. They are firm, rubbery nodules that may continue to enlarge for years (see **Figure 2**).

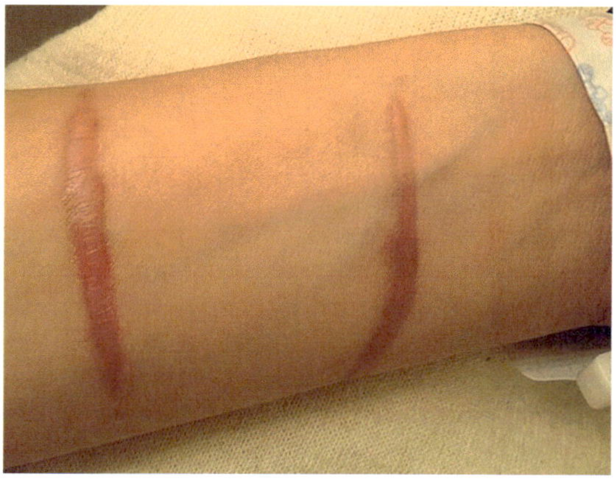

Figure 1.
Hypertrophic scars present as raised, erythematous, and firm lesions that remain confined within the original wound boundaries.

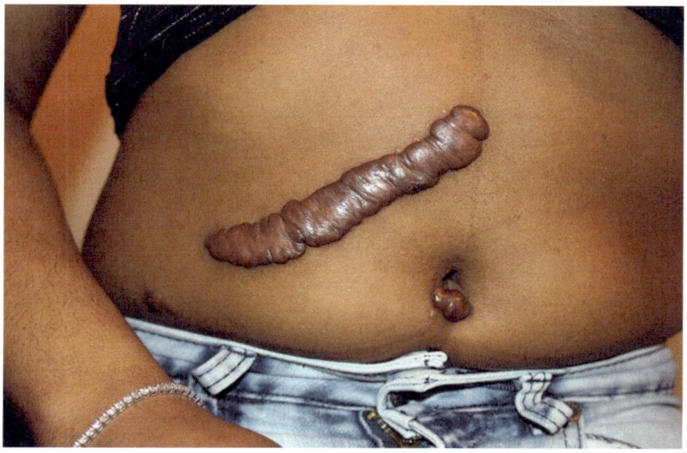

Figure 2.
Keloids present as firm, rubbery nodules that often extend beyond the original borders of the wound.

Histologically, keloids demonstrate thick, hyalinized collagen bundles arranged haphazardly, reduced apoptosis of fibroblasts, and sustained overexpression of profibrotic cytokines such as TGF-β and CTGF [24, 25].

Although less common after burns than hypertrophic scars, keloids can arise in susceptible individuals – particularly those with darker Fitzpatrick skin types (IV–VI) and a family history of keloid formation [24]. Common sites include the chest, shoulders, jawline, and earlobes, where skin tension is high. Genetic predisposition, chronic inflammation, and delayed wound healing contribute to their development.

Keloids are notoriously resistant to treatment, with high recurrence rates following excision alone. Combination therapy – such as intralesional corticosteroids, 5-fluorouracil, cryotherapy, radiation, or laser therapy – offers improved control [26, 27]. Their aesthetic impact, along with symptoms of pain or itching, can significantly affect quality of life, underscoring the need for preventive strategies in high-risk patients.

3.3 Contractures

Contractures arise when excessive myofibroblast-mediated contraction and collagen cross-linking reduce the pliability of the skin across joints or flexural creases (see **Figure 3**) [28]. Unlike hypertrophic scars or keloids, which are primarily cosmetic or localized, contractures produce mechanical restriction and functional disability. They are most pronounced following deep burns in regions of high mobility, such as the neck, axilla, elbows, and hands.

Patients present with a limited range of motion, skin tethering, and deformity of underlying structures. In severe cases, joint ankylosis and growth restriction may occur in pediatric populations [29]. Early physical and occupational therapy, splinting, and timely surgical release are essential for restoring function.

4. Conservative and nonsurgical management

Conservative management forms the cornerstone of burn scar therapy, aiming to prevent hypertrophic scarring, promote optimal wound remodeling, and maintain functional mobility. These modalities are most effective when initiated early – ideally during the proliferative phase of wound healing – and continued throughout scar maturation [30, 31]. Nonsurgical strategies act by modulating the mechanical, biochemical, and inflammatory cues that perpetuate fibrosis, complementing procedural or surgical interventions when required.

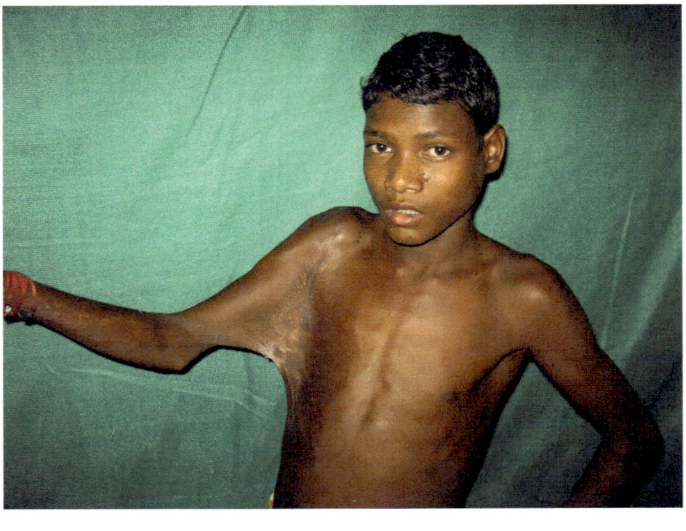

Figure 3.
Contractures present with limited range of motion, skin tethering, and deformity of underlying structures across joints affected by a previous burn.

4.1 Pressure therapy

Pressure garment therapy (PGT) remains one of the most established modalities in burn scar prevention. Continuous mechanical compression (15–30 mmHg) is believed to decrease dermal blood flow, tissue oxygen tension, and collagen synthesis while realigning collagen fibers parallel to the skin surface (see **Figure 4**) [32, 33]. This reduction in perfusion limits fibroblast proliferation and downregulates TGF-β activity, thereby reducing scar hypertrophy.

Garments are custom-fitted and typically worn 23 hours per day for 6–18 months, depending on scar maturity. Effectiveness is highest when therapy begins immediately after wound epithelialization. Adherence remains a challenge due to discomfort, heat, and pruritus, particularly in pediatric patients.

While randomized trials show variable benefits, meta-analyses suggest that PGT modestly improves scar height and pliability, particularly when combined with silicone therapy or massage [32, 34]. Optimal pressure levels, wear duration, and compliance remain areas of ongoing research.

4.2 Silicone gel and sheets

Silicone therapy – either as occlusive sheets or topical gels – is a first-line, noninvasive treatment shown to reduce scar erythema, thickness, and pruritus [35, 36]. The mechanism is multifactorial: occlusion and hydration of the stratum corneum reduce transepidermal water loss, restore barrier function, and suppress mast cell–mediated cytokine release [37, 38]. Additionally, silicone generates a static electric field that may influence fibroblast activity and collagen alignment [39].

Silicone sheets are applied directly over healed skin for 12–24 hours daily and maintained for at least 2–3 months. Silicone gels provide an alternative for irregular surfaces, such as the face or joints. Side effects are minimal, primarily limited to mild maceration or rash.

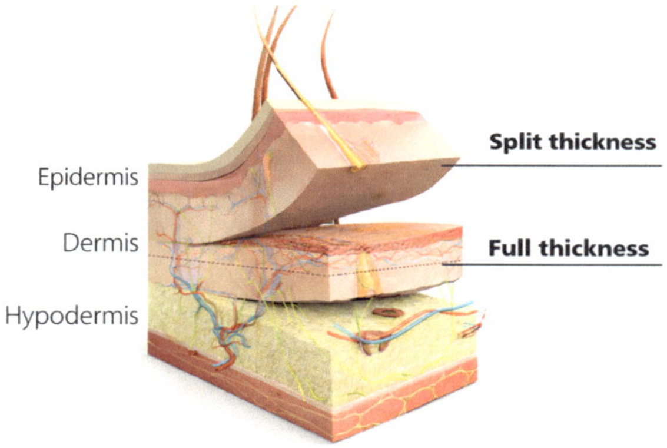

Figure 4.
Cross-sectional schematic of skin demonstrating the epidermis, dermis, and hypodermis with comparative graft harvest planes. In a split-thickness skin graft (STSG), the epidermis and a portion of the superficial dermis are elevated, leaving behind deeper dermal elements within the donor site. In a full-thickness skin graft (FTSG), the epidermis and the entire dermis are harvested en bloc, with the dissection plane immediately superficial to the subcutaneous fat.

Multiple systematic reviews, including Cochrane analyses, affirm moderate evidence for silicone's benefit in scar flattening and softening [40]. It remains the gold standard adjunct to pressure therapy in both the prevention and early treatment of hypertrophic scars.

4.3 Massage therapy and moisturization

Scar massage enhances pliability, reduces pruritus, and alleviates discomfort by disrupting adhesions, improving local circulation, and modulating mechanotransduction pathways within fibroblasts [41]. Regular mechanical stimulation may attenuate excessive collagen deposition and promote reorganization of ECM fibers [28, 42].

Massage is initiated after complete epithelialization and is performed 2–3 times daily for 5–10 minutes using circular or linear motions with emollients or silicone-based gels. Moisturization complements massage by reducing transepidermal water loss and preventing fissuring, which can trigger inflammation.

Although clinical studies are heterogeneous, consistent findings support improved elasticity, reduced pain, and decreased pruritus with structured massage programs as part of multidisciplinary rehabilitation [43].

4.4 Physical and occupational therapy

Physical and occupational therapy are essential to prevent contracture formation, preserve range of motion, and maintain functional alignment during the healing process. Stretching counteracts myofibroblast-mediated contraction by applying controlled mechanical stress, which promotes collagen realignment and elongation [42].

Therapists employ passive and active range-of-motion exercises, splinting, and positioning techniques to counteract deforming forces. Early mobilization – within days of graft healing – is critical to prevent joint stiffness. Pressure garments and splints are often used synergistically during exercise to optimize outcomes.

Clinical trials consistently demonstrate that early, intensive rehabilitation reduces contracture severity and improves long-term function, emphasizing the role of therapy as a preventive rather than a corrective measure [44].

4.5 Pharmacologic topical and intralesional agents

4.5.1 Topical corticosteroids

Corticosteroids reduce fibroblast proliferation, collagen synthesis, and inflammatory cytokine release [45]. Although primarily used as intralesional injections for established scars, topical preparations (e.g., hydrocortisone, clobetasol) may be beneficial for pruritus and erythema in early scars [46].

4.5.2 Onion extract, vitamin E, and emerging topicals

Commercial preparations containing *Allium cepa* extract, tocopherol (vitamin E), and heparin have been marketed to improve scar appearance, though clinical evidence remains limited and inconsistent [47, 48]. Research continues into topical formulations incorporating TGF-β inhibitors, interferons, and botulinum toxin A for noninvasive scar modulation.

5. Laser and energy-based therapies

5.1 Overview and principles of laser therapy

Laser therapy has become an integral component of modern burn scar management, providing a means of selectively remodeling scar tissue through controlled photothermal injury. The fundamental concept underlying laser treatment is selective photothermolysis, whereby specific wavelengths of light are absorbed by target chromophores – most commonly oxyhemoglobin or water – resulting in localized thermal effects while minimizing collateral tissue injury. By precisely modulating light-tissue interactions, lasers can influence vascularity, pigmentation, collagen architecture, and overall pliability of burn scars [49].

Lasers used in scar management are broadly categorized as ablative or nonablative based on their depth and mechanism of tissue interaction. Ablative lasers, such as carbon dioxide (CO_2, 10,600 nm) and erbium:yttrium aluminum garnet (Er:YAG, 2,940 nm), target water in the skin and vaporize microcolumns of tissue to induce thermal coagulation in the dermis, thereby stimulating neocollagenesis and reorganization of collagen bundles. The introduction of fractional laser technology, which delivers energy in microscopic treatment zones (MTZs) interspersed with untreated skin, has markedly improved safety, recovery time, and the feasibility of treating large burn scars. Nonablative lasers, including 1,540–1,550 nm systems, remodel dermal collagen without ablating the epidermis.

In burn care, laser therapy serves two principal purposes: early intervention to modulate inflammation and vascularity in immature scars, and later intervention to remodel established fibrosis, reduce pruritus and pain, and improve functional mobility. The most widely used systems in clinical burn scar management include pulsed dye lasers (PDL), fractional CO_2 lasers, Er:YAG lasers, and nonablative fractional devices, often employed in a complementary fashion within multidisciplinary treatment protocols.

5.2 Pulsed dye laser

The PDL (585–595 nm) was the first device shown to significantly improve hypertrophic burn scars by targeting oxyhemoglobin in hypervascular tissue [49]. Absorption of this wavelength leads to selective photothermolysis of abnormal microvasculature, resulting in reduced erythema, edema, and inflammatory signaling. The PDL therapy also downregulates TGF-β and other profibrotic cytokines, thereby modulating fibroblast activity and collagen deposition [50].

The PDL is particularly effective during the early, immature phase of burn scar formation, when vascularity and erythema are most pronounced. Treatment is typically initiated after complete epithelialization, using fluences of 6–8 J/cm^2, pulse durations of 0.45–1.5 ms, and dynamic cooling to minimize epidermal damage.

Clinical evidence strongly supports its efficacy. A 2025 multicenter randomized controlled trial – the Early Laser for Burn Scar Study (ELABS) – demonstrated that the early addition of PDL to standard care significantly improved overall scar quality and patient-reported quality of life compared with standard therapy alone [51]. Other prospective studies and systematic reviews have consistently reported improvements in Vancouver Scar Scale (VSS) scores, particularly in the vascularity and pliability domains, as well as reductions in pruritus and pain [52]. Adverse effects are typically mild and transient, consisting primarily of purpura and posttreatment erythema that resolve within days [53].

5.3 Fractional CO_2 laser

The fractional carbon dioxide (CO_2) laser (10,600 nm) has emerged as the workhorse for the treatment of mature, thick, or contracted burn scars. By creating an array of microscopic ablation columns surrounded by zones of thermal coagulation, the CO_2 laser induces controlled dermal injury that stimulates collagen remodeling, elastin neogenesis, and soft-tissue relaxation. The result is a gradual improvement in texture, pliability, and range of motion, particularly across joints or areas of contracture.

Ablative fractional CO_2 laser therapy has demonstrated measurable functional and symptomatic benefits in burn survivors. In a randomized controlled trial summarized in a 2019 evidence review, CO_2-treated burn scars exhibited significant reductions in pruritus and pain compared with untreated control sites [54]. Multiple cohort studies have also shown improvements in VSS parameters, including height, pliability, and vascularity, as well as objective gains in joint range of motion following serial treatments [55, 56]. Typical treatment parameters include energies of 30–60 mJ per microbeam, densities of 5–20%, and intervals of 8–12 weeks between sessions.

The safety profile of fractional CO_2 treatment is favorable, though transient erythema, edema, or pigmentary alterations may occur, particularly in darker skin types [57]. These risks can be mitigated with conservative energy settings and pretreatment counseling.

5.4 Fractional Er:YAG laser

The Er:YAG laser (2,940 nm) operates at a wavelength with even higher absorption by water than CO_2, producing more superficial ablation with less thermal coagulation. This results in shorter healing times and a lower risk of pigmentary change [58]. Fractional Er:YAG is especially suitable for facial scars, thin grafted skin, and pediatric populations, where downtime and thermal injury must be minimized.

Comparative studies of Er:YAG and CO_2 lasers in burn scar management have demonstrated that both modalities yield significant improvements in scar thickness, elasticity, and pigmentation [59]. However, CO_2 lasers tend to achieve greater soft-tissue release in deeper or more fibrotic scars, whereas Er:YAG offers faster recovery and superior textural refinement [60]. In recent trials, Er:YAG therapy improved validated scar assessment scores in both immature and mature scars after a series of three to five sessions spaced 4–8 weeks apart [61].

5.5 Nonablative fractional lasers (1,540–1,550 nm)

Nonablative fractional lasers deliver mid-infrared light that penetrates the dermis while preserving the epidermis. The resulting sublethal thermal injury promotes collagen remodeling through fibroblast activation without creating open wounds, making this modality particularly appealing to patients with large treatment areas, higher Fitzpatrick skin types, or medical comorbidities that preclude aggressive therapy [62, 63].

In a prospective study using a 1,550-nm fractional laser for burn scars, 90% of patients demonstrated at least mild improvement, and 60% achieved moderate to excellent results after three sessions, with minimal downtime or adverse events [64]. Nonablative systems are often employed as adjuncts to other modalities – such as after PDL for vascular normalization or alternating with CO_2 laser for incremental remodeling – thereby expanding therapeutic versatility across diverse scar presentations [65].

5.6 Long-pulsed Nd:YAG and intense pulsed light

The long-pulsed Nd:YAG laser (1,064 nm) targets deeper vascular structures than the PDL and can penetrate more fibrotic tissue. Although evidence in burn-specific populations remains limited, it may benefit thicker or more mature scars with persistent erythema [66].

Intense pulsed light (IPL) systems emit a broad spectrum of light (515–1,200 nm), filtered to target oxyhemoglobin and melanin. The IPL offers outcomes comparable to PDL in reducing erythema and vascularity, but with a lower incidence of purpura. In a 2023 comparative review, IPL achieved similar reductions in scar redness and texture in hypertrophic burn scars, making it a practical alternative when PDL is unavailable or when patients prefer a less bruising modality [67].

5.7 Combined and sequential laser approaches

The multifactorial pathophysiology of burn scarring often warrants combination therapy to address vascular, textural, and mechanical components simultaneously. Sequential or concurrent use of PDL (for vascular modulation) and fractional CO_2 or Er:YAG (for remodeling) has demonstrated superior improvement in scar height, pliability, and pigmentation compared with monotherapy. Combination approaches also allow for lower fluences and reduced treatment intervals, minimizing side effects while maximizing outcomes. Ablative fractional lasers may also be paired with topical or intralesional agents, such as corticosteroids or 5-fluorouracil, through the principle of laser-assisted drug delivery, enhancing tissue penetration and local efficacy.

5.8 Clinical integration and treatment timing

The timing of laser intervention is critical to the outcome. Early vascular lasers (PDL or IPL) are best employed during the proliferative phase – typically within 1–3 months of wound closure – to suppress inflammation, vascular proliferation, and fibroblast hyperactivity. In contrast, fractional ablative lasers (CO_2 or Er:YAG) are indicated for mature, stable scars to induce long-term remodeling and improve pliability and function. Corticosteroid injections are often used in conjunction with laser therapy, as they directly inhibit fibroblast proliferation and collagen synthesis, thereby augmenting laser-mediated remodeling and reducing hypertrophic progression or recurrence.

For severe contractures or rigid scars crossing joints, fractional CO_2 laser treatment can be strategically combined with physical therapy to enhance soft-tissue release and maintain gains in range of motion. Patients should be counseled regarding the need for multiple sessions – commonly 3 to 6 – and the gradual nature of improvement.

6. Surgical management

Although advances in conservative, pharmacologic, and laser-based modalities have significantly reduced the burden of postburn fibrosis, surgical management remains the cornerstone for treating scars that cause functional limitation, contracture, or severe aesthetic deformity. Surgical intervention is particularly indicated when mature scar tissue restricts motion across joints, distorts anatomic landmarks, or produces disabling contractures that impair daily activity. The overarching goals of surgery are to release pathologic scar tissue, restore mobility, reestablish contour, and resurface the defect with tissue of adequate elasticity and durability. Successful outcomes depend not only on the surgical technique itself but also on meticulous preoperative planning, timing of intervention, and comprehensive postoperative rehabilitation.

In most cases, surgical reconstruction is deferred until the scar has matured – typically six to 12 months after injury – when erythema, vascularity, and inflammation have subsided. However, early release may be necessary if contracture formation interferes with growth or function, such as periocular ectropion causing corneal exposure or microstomia impairing oral intake.

6.1 Excision and grafting

Excision and grafting form the foundation of burn scar reconstruction. The technique involves excising fibrotic tissue to restore motion and replacing it with healthy, pliable skin. The goal is to provide durable coverage that maintains elasticity, minimizes recurrence, and improves aesthetic outcomes.

Surgical excision must extend through the full thickness of the scar into viable tissue with adequate vascularity. Incomplete excision leaves behind fibrotic remnants that can perpetuate contracture. After achieving hemostasis, the wound bed is resurfaced with an autologous skin graft – either split-thickness skin graft (STSGs) or full-thickness skin graft (FTSGs) – depending on the size of the defect, depth of release, and aesthetic priorities.

6.1.1 Split-thickness skin grafts

Split-thickness skin grafts, harvested at 0.012–0.018 inches, include the epidermis and superficial dermis (see **Figure 4**). They are technically straightforward to harvest, allow for large-area coverage, and have reliable graft take due to their lower metabolic demands. However, STSGs are prone to secondary contraction, making them less ideal for high-mobility regions such as the neck, axilla, or hands [68]. The resulting surface may also differ in pigmentation and texture from adjacent normal skin.

DOI: http://dx.doi.org/10.5772/intechopen.1015801

6.1.2 Full-thickness skin grafts

Full-thickness skin grafts incorporate both the epidermis and the entire dermis, offering superior elasticity, pigmentation match, and resistance to recontracture. The FTSGs are especially indicated for functionally and cosmetically sensitive areas, including the face, eyelids, and digits. Their take rates are lower than those of STSGs on poorly vascularized beds, necessitating precise hemostasis and immobile contact during the early postoperative period. Donor sites – such as the groin, supraclavicular region, or postauricular skin – can usually be closed primarily, limiting donor morbidity.

6.1.3 Technique, postoperative care, and outcomes

After scar excision, the graft is contoured to fit the defect and secured with fine sutures or staples. Immobilization using tie-over dressings or negative-pressure wound therapy (NPWT) helps ensure graft adherence by removing interstitial fluid and improving neovascularization. Postoperatively, pressure garments, silicone sheeting, and early physiotherapy are essential to prevent recurrence. Regular monitoring for hematoma, infection, or partial graft loss is critical, as these complications may lead to secondary fibrosis.

Numerous studies have documented functional and aesthetic improvements following grafting procedures [69]. Full-thickness grafts provide the most durable outcomes, whereas split-thickness grafts may require subsequent revisions. Despite successful release, recurrence of contracture has been reported in up to 20–30% of cases when postoperative rehabilitation is suboptimal [70]. Integrating fractional CO_2 laser therapy during follow-up can further enhance pliability and texture in grafted areas.

6.2 Tissue arrangement techniques

Tissue arrangement techniques form the foundation of surgical management for scar contractures, allowing lengthening, redirection, and redistribution of scar tension while preserving well-vascularized tissue. These techniques are broadly categorized into local, regional, and free (autologous) tissue reconstruction, with local tissue arrangement representing the most commonly employed and conceptually important approach for contracture release.

6.2.1 Local tissue arrangement techniques

Local tissue rearrangement utilizes adjacent skin and subcutaneous tissue to release contractures while maintaining an optimal color, texture, thickness, and sensibility match. These techniques are particularly effective for linear or band-like contractures of the neck, hand, axilla, perioral region, and flexion creases and demonstrate superior resistance to recontracture compared with skin grafting alone [71].

6.2.1.1 Geometric lengthening plasties

Geometric lengthening plasties are based on the transposition of triangular or polygonal flaps to achieve lengthening along the axis of maximal contracture and to reorient scars along relaxed skin tension lines.

Z-plasty remains the most versatile and commonly employed technique. The central limb is aligned with the line of greatest tension, while the lateral limbs generate theoretical lengthening proportional to their angle. Variations include serial Z-plasty for long linear contractures, double-opposing (four-flap) Z-plasty, and the five-flap ("jumping man") Z-plasty, which provide increased lengthening and are particularly useful for severe web-space or commissural contractures (see **Figure 5**). Broken or irregular Z-plasties may be used to disrupt long linear scars and reduce recurrent contractures [71, 72].

6.2.1.2 Advancement techniques

Advancement flaps mobilize tissue directly into the defect following contracture release (see **Figure 6**). Straight-line and bipedicled advancement flaps preserve dual blood supply and are useful for linear bands, while V–Y advancement flaps are especially effective for focal contractures involving the oral commissure, axilla, digits, or flexion creases. These techniques provide reliable lengthening while maintaining robust vascularity and are frequently combined with geometric plasties in more complex reconstructions [71].

6.2.1.3 Rotational flaps

Rotational flaps redistribute tension by rotating a semicircular flap into the defect created by scar release (see **Figure 7**). Classic rotation flaps, rotation–advancement flaps, and crescentic rotational flaps are useful when straight-line advancement would result in excessive tension or distortion of adjacent anatomic units. These flaps are particularly valuable in the neck and axilla, where broader arcs of rotation are required [71, 73].

6.2.1.4 Transposition flaps

Transposition flaps transfer tissue across an intervening area of intact skin to resurface the defect (see **Figure 8**). Common examples include rhomboid (Limberg), bilobed, and hatchet flaps. In contracture reconstruction, these flaps are most useful when tissue must be recruited from a nonadjacent direction to optimize tension vectors and contour [72].

6.2.1.5 Local perforator-based flaps

Advances in perforator flap design have expanded the role of local tissue rearrangement in contracture surgery. Perforator island flaps and propeller flaps allow rotation or advancement of thin, pliable tissue based on a single perforator, extending flap reach while minimizing donor-site morbidity. These flaps are increasingly used for cervical, axillary, and extremity contractures and offer improved durability compared to traditional random-pattern flaps [73].

6.2.2 Regional flap reconstruction

When local tissue rearrangement is insufficient due to extensive scarring or tissue deficiency, regional flaps provide well-vascularized coverage over larger areas.

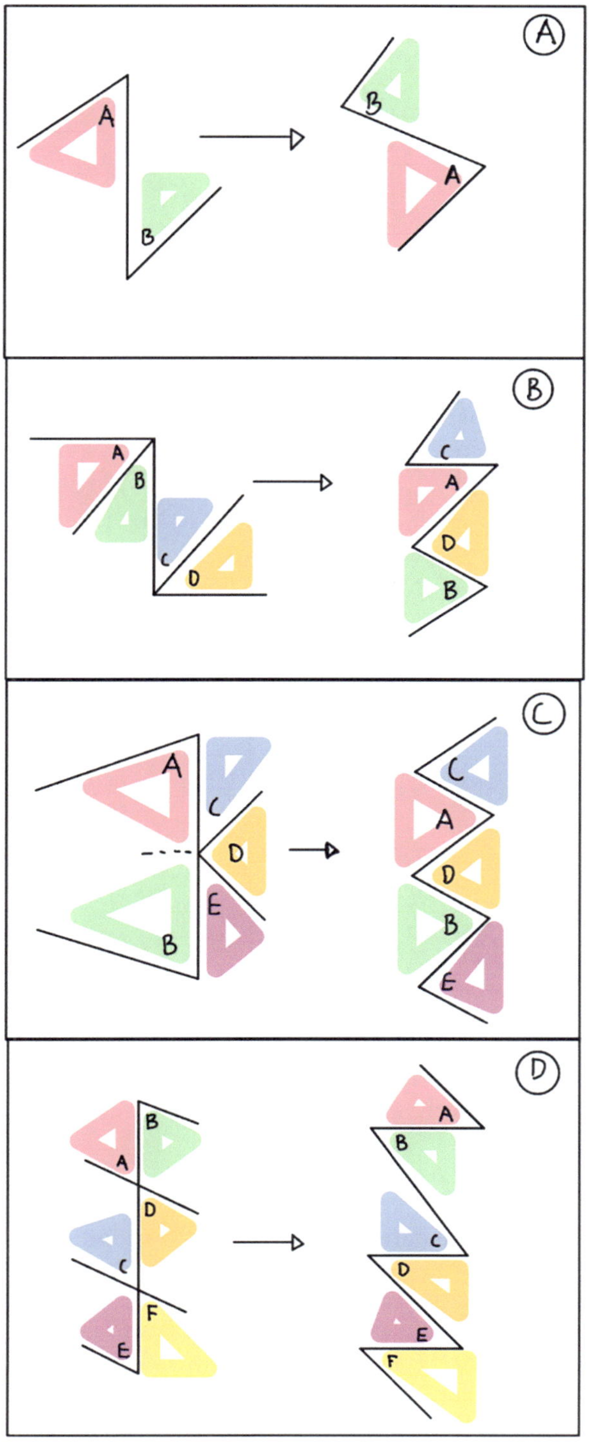

Figure 5.
Schematic of (a) single Z-plasty, (b) four-flap Z-plasty, (c) five-flap Z-plasty, and (d) multiple aligned Z-plasties.

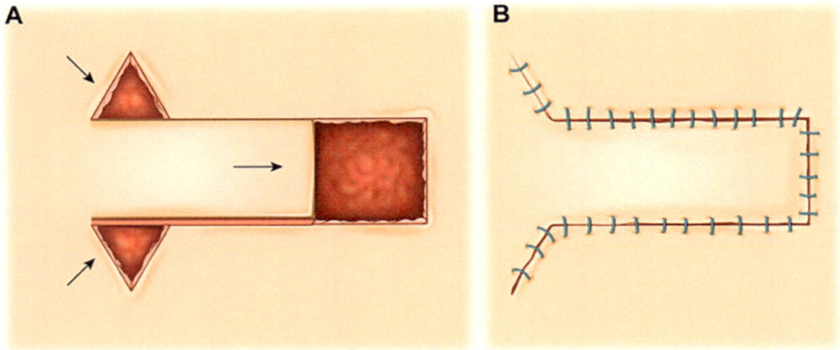

Figure 6.
Schematic of a V–Y advancement flap.

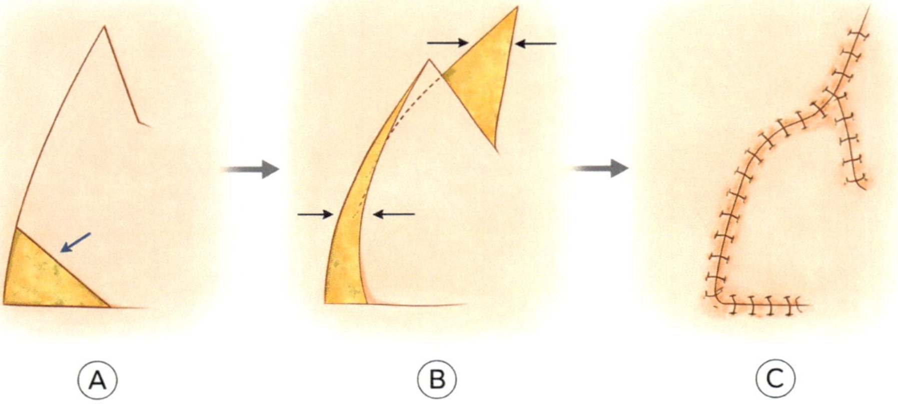

Figure 7.
Schematic of a rotational flap.

Commonly utilized regional flaps include the deltopectoral, trapezius, and parascapular flaps, particularly for axillary and cervical contractures [71].

6.2.3 Free (autologous) tissue reconstruction

Free tissue transfer is indicated for large, recurrent, or severe contractures when local and regional options are unavailable or inadequate (see **Figure 9**). Common free flaps include the anterolateral thigh (ALT), radial forearm, and groin flaps, which provide thin, pliable tissue suitable for areas of motion. Flap-based reconstruction offers superior resistance to recontracture compared with grafts, particularly across joints and dynamic regions [71–73].

6.3 Tissue expansion and contracture release

Tissue expansion leverages the skin's inherent viscoelastic properties and regenerative capacity to create new tissue for reconstruction. By gradually stretching

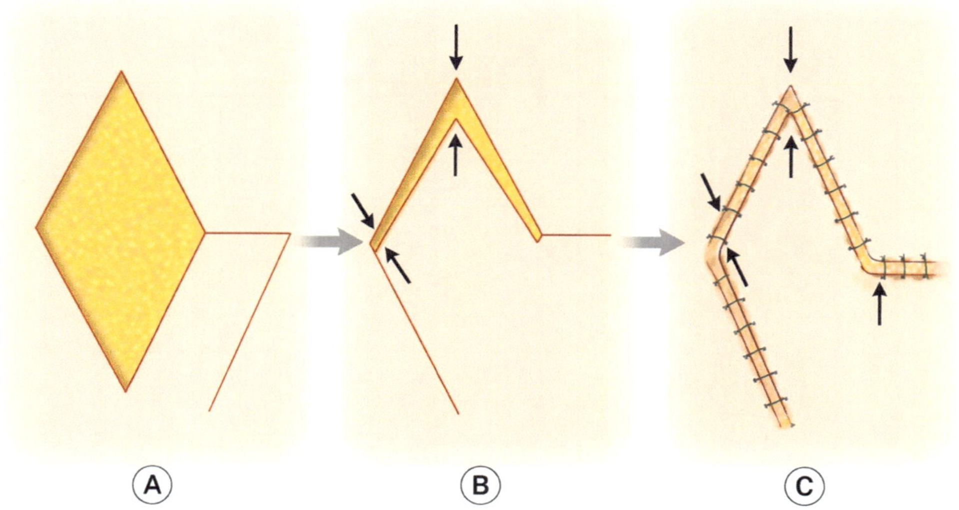

Figure 8.
Schematic of a transposition flap.

the skin adjacent to a burn scar, surgeons can generate additional tissue that matches the surrounding area in texture, color, and thickness. This method is particularly valuable in the face, scalp, neck, and upper chest, where tissue match is critical for both function and aesthetics.

A silicone expander is placed in the subcutaneous plane near the scar to be reconstructed. After wound healing and stabilization, gradual expansion begins, usually within two to three weeks postinsertion. Saline is injected through a remote port weekly or biweekly, with incremental increases of 10–15% of the expander's volume per session. Overexpansion – often 25–30% beyond the desired surface area – is performed to compensate for recoil once the expander is removed (see **Figure 10**).

After sufficient tissue has been generated, the expander is removed, the scar is excised or the contracture released, and the newly expanded tissue is advanced or rotated into the defect. Expanded tissue maintains its vascular supply and exhibits minimal secondary contraction.

The principal advantage of tissue expansion is that it produces replacement tissue identical to the recipient site, offering excellent color, texture, and thickness match. It avoids additional donor-site scars and provides durable results with minimal long-term contraction. However, tissue expansion requires multiple procedures and prolonged treatment duration, often spanning several months. Complications such as infection, extrusion, expander rupture, or hematoma occur in up to 10–15% of cases. Successful outcomes demand meticulous technique, aseptic handling, and patient adherence to the expansion schedule.

Tissue expansion is often integrated into staged reconstructive plans, combining expansion with contracture release and flap or graft coverage. This comprehensive approach is particularly effective in reconstructing large cervical or facial burn deformities. After expansion-based reconstruction, adjunctive therapies – such as

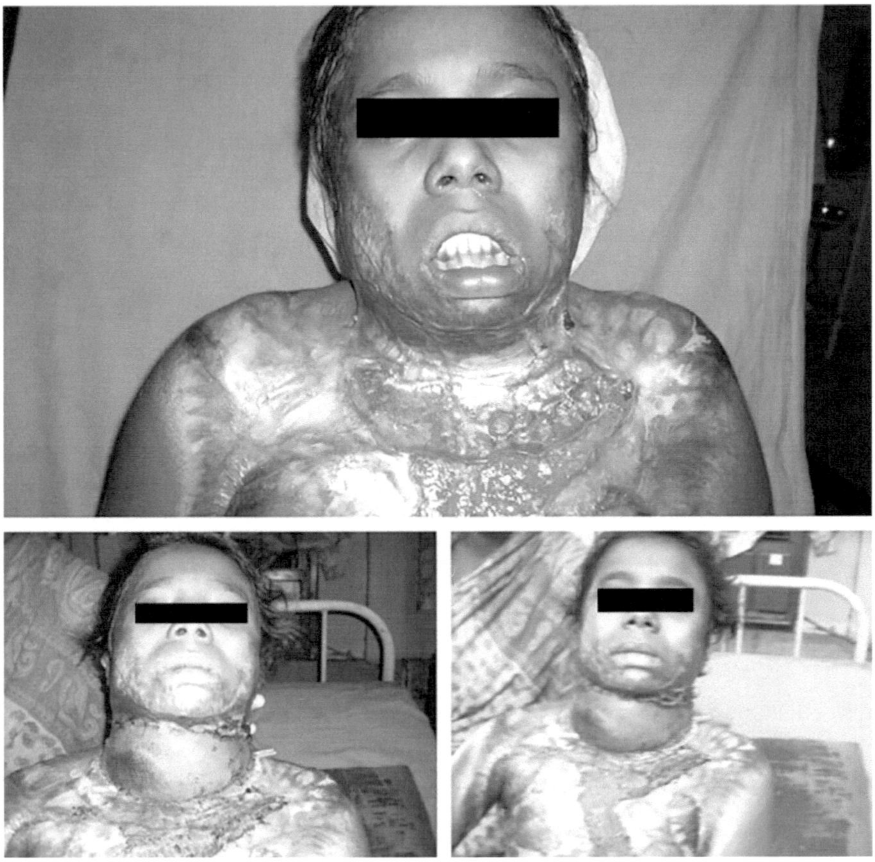

Figure 9.
Preoperative clinical photograph (top) demonstrates severe anterior neck postburn scar contracture with mentosternal tethering and restricted cervical extension. Following contracture release, reconstruction was performed using a free anterolateral thigh (ALT) flap. Postoperative views (bottom left and right) demonstrate successful resurfacing of the anterior neck with improved contour and restoration of cervical extension after flap inset.

laser resurfacing and physical therapy – enhance the contour, texture, and mobility of the newly transferred skin.

7. Regenerative and emerging therapies

Over the past decade, a paradigm shift has emerged in burn scar management – from traditional excisional and reconstructive techniques aimed at replacing scarred tissue to regenerative approaches designed to restore native skin architecture and function. These novel therapies seek to modulate inflammation, promote angiogenesis, and stimulate cellular regeneration, moving beyond scar revision to scar reversal.

Among the most promising innovations are autologous fat grafting, stem cell–based therapies, bioengineered scaffolds, and PBM. Collectively, these modalities exploit advances in molecular biology, tissue engineering, and regenerative medicine to improve both functional and aesthetic outcomes for burn survivors.

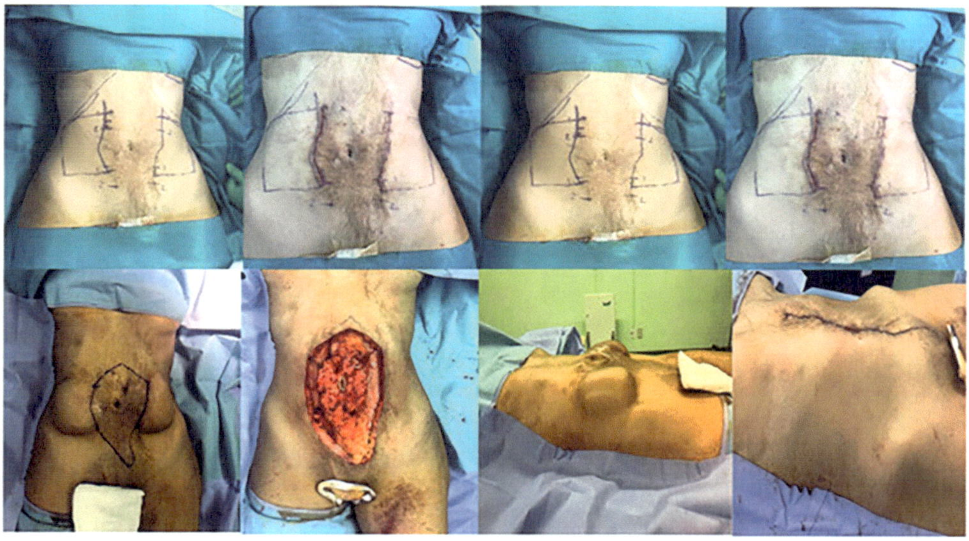

Figure 10.
Clinical photographs demonstrating staged bilateral subcutaneous tissue expansion adjacent to the umbilicus for reconstruction of a contracted periumbilical scar. Tissue expanders were placed lateral to the umbilicus and serially inflated to recruit adjacent abdominal skin. Following adequate expansion, the scar was excised, the expanders were removed, and the expanded skin was advanced to resurface the defect and restore abdominal contour.

7.1 Fat grafting

Autologous fat grafting, or lipofilling, has gained widespread use as a minimally invasive approach for improving burn scar pliability, contour, and quality. Adipose tissue is not merely a filler – it is a rich reservoir of adipose-derived stem cells (ASCs), growth factors, and ECM components that facilitate neovascularization, fibroblast modulation, and dermal regeneration.

Injected adipocytes release paracrine mediators, such as vascular endothelial growth factor (VEGF), hepatocyte growth factor (HGF), and basic fibroblast growth factor (bFGF), which enhance tissue perfusion and reduce inflammation [74, 75]. The ASCs, in particular, have been shown to downregulate TGF-β1 expression, thereby mitigating fibrosis and promoting the deposition of more organized collagen [76].

Fat grafting is performed using low-pressure liposuction (e.g., Coleman technique) to harvest adipose tissue, typically from the abdomen or thighs. The lipoaspirate is processed via centrifugation or filtration to remove oil and debris, and microdroplets are injected in multiple planes within the scarred tissue. Fractional CO_2 laser pretreatment is sometimes used to create microchannels, enhancing graft integration. The procedure may require serial sessions spaced 3–6 months apart to achieve optimal outcomes, as partial resorption (20–40%) is common.

Multiple clinical studies demonstrate meaningful improvement in scar pliability, pain, and pigmentation following autologous fat grafting in burn scars. A meta-analysis reported significant enhancements in VSS and Patient and Observer Scar Assessment Scale (POSAS) scores, as well as reduced pruritus and stiffness [77]. Imaging studies using ultrasound and histologic evaluation reveal increased dermal thickness, neovascularization, and partial restoration of the subcutaneous plane [78]. Fat grafting is especially valuable for atrophic or adherent scars, perioral and periorbital contractures, and contour irregularities after graft or flap reconstruction.

Challenges include unpredictable resorption, donor-site morbidity, and variable cell survival. Processing techniques, such as nanofat or stromal vascular fraction (SVF)–enriched fat grafting, may improve retention and biologic activity, though standardization and long-term data remain areas of ongoing research.

7.2 Stem cell therapy

Stem cell–based therapy represents a frontier in regenerative burn care. Several cell populations have demonstrated antifibrotic, angiogenic, and immunomodulatory properties, including ASCs, bone marrow–derived mesenchymal stem cells (BM-MSCs), and induced pluripotent stem cells (iPSCs).

These cells secrete cytokines such as IL-10, VEGF, and epidermal growth factor (EGF), which regulate fibroblast proliferation, promote reepithelialization, and attenuate scar contracture [79, 80]. Rather than differentiating directly into skin cells, stem cells largely act through paracrine signaling, altering the wound microenvironment to favor regenerative over fibrotic healing [81].

Despite encouraging results, stem cell therapy faces barriers to widespread clinical adoption. These include regulatory hurdles, variability in cell isolation protocols, and uncertainties surrounding long-term safety and engraftment. Future strategies may involve gene-edited MSCs or cell-free therapies utilizing exosomes derived from stem cells, which deliver regenerative microRNAs and growth factors without the risks of live-cell implantation.

7.3 Biomaterials and scaffolds

Bioengineered materials and scaffolds are designed to replicate the structural and biochemical properties of native dermis, guiding cellular migration and matrix deposition during tissue repair. Their use in burn scar management aims to restore elasticity, improve graft integration, and minimize fibrosis by providing an optimal microenvironment for regenerative healing.

Natural scaffolds – such as collagen, fibrin, chitosan, and hyaluronic acid–based matrices – offer inherent biocompatibility and bioactivity that support fibroblast and keratinocyte adhesion. Commercially available bilayer dermal substitutes, composed of collagen–glycosaminoglycan matrices paired with a temporary epidermal layer, have shown improvements in scar quality and reductions in postburn contracture rates [82]. In contrast, synthetic scaffolds made from polymers like polylactic-co-glycolic acid (PLGA) and polycaprolactone (PCL) provide customizable mechanical properties and predictable degradation. These materials can also be adapted for 3D bioprinting, allowing for patient-specific fabrication of dermal templates and composite graft constructs.

The integration of biomaterials with stem cells or growth factors represents an evolving frontier in regenerative burn care. Stem cell–seeded scaffolds enhance angiogenesis and modulate inflammation, while controlled-release systems delivering VEGF, TGF-β inhibitors, or platelet-derived growth factor (PDGF) provide sustained biochemical signaling to guide organized tissue formation [83].

Preclinical studies have demonstrated that composite scaffolds seeded with ASCs can regenerate skin containing adnexal structures and reduce scar contracture compared with acellular grafts alone [84]. While the results are promising, challenges remain regarding scaffold integration, immunogenicity, and cost. Long-term data on functional durability are limited, and most applications currently occur within tertiary or experimental settings.

7.4 Photobiomodulation

Photobiomodulation, also known as low-level light therapy (LLLT), utilizes nonthermal light energy in the red (630–700 nm) or near-infrared (780–950 nm) spectrum to stimulate cellular metabolism and tissue repair. The PBM acts primarily through the activation of cytochrome c oxidase in the mitochondrial respiratory chain, leading to increased ATP production, modulation of reactive oxygen species, and upregulation of transcription factors that govern cell proliferation and cytokine release [85, 86].

In burn scars, PBM has been shown to reduce inflammation, enhance collagen organization, and improve microcirculation [87]. The therapy promotes the transition of fibroblasts to a more quiescent phenotype while stimulating endothelial proliferation and angiogenesis. Additionally, PBM attenuates TGF-β1 and α-SMA expression, thereby reducing myofibroblast activity and contracture potential [88, 89].

Clinical studies demonstrate that PBM can improve pain, pruritus, and scar pliability in both hypertrophic and postsurgical scars [49]. A randomized controlled trial using 808-nm diode laser therapy applied twice weekly for eight weeks showed significant improvements in POSAS and VSS scores compared with standard care alone [90]. Other trials using red LED light (635 nm) have reported accelerated healing and improved scar appearance following grafting or laser resurfacing [91].

The PBM is typically administered 2–3 times per week for several weeks, with fluences ranging from 3 to 6 J/cm^2 per session. Adverse effects are rare and limited to transient warmth or erythema. PBM is increasingly used as an adjunct to surgical and laser-based therapies. Postlaser PBM can enhance re-epithelialization and reduce downtime, while preconditioning with PBM may improve graft survival by enhancing local perfusion [92]. Its low cost, safety, and noninvasive nature make it a promising addition to multidisciplinary scar management programs.

8. Multidisciplinary and rehabilitation approaches

Optimal burn scar management extends far beyond the operating room or clinic. Achieving durable, functional, and aesthetic recovery requires a comprehensive, multidisciplinary approach that addresses the biological, mechanical, and psychosocial dimensions of healing. The modern standard of care emphasizes early and continuous collaboration among surgeons, physical/occupational therapists, nurses, psychologists, and social workers. This team-based strategy ensures that scar management is proactive, not reactive – anticipating complications and guiding patients through all phases of recovery, from acute wound closure to long-term rehabilitation.

8.1 The multidisciplinary burn team

The multidisciplinary burn team operates as a coordinated unit, in which each member contributes specialized expertise toward a shared goal: restoring function, comfort, and self-image (see **Figure 11**).

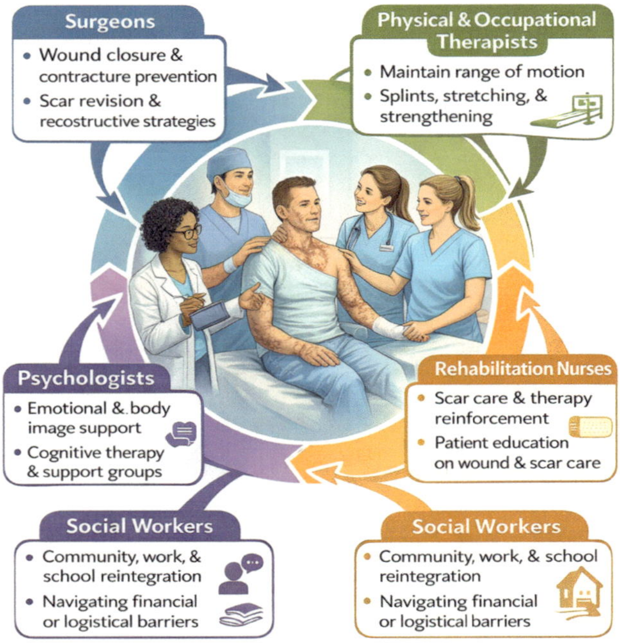

Figure 11.
Illustration of the coordinated, multidisciplinary approach to burn rehabilitation.

- Surgeons focus on wound closure, contracture prevention, and reconstructive strategies while coordinating long-term scar revision when indicated.

- Physical and occupational therapists maintain the range of motion, prevent contractures, and promote functional independence through stretching, splinting, and strengthening programs.

- Rehabilitation nurses provide ongoing wound and scar care, patient education, and reinforcement of therapy regimens.

- Psychologists address the profound emotional and body image challenges that accompany visible scarring, employing cognitive behavioral therapy and support groups to enhance coping.

- Social workers assist with reintegration into community, work, and school environments, as well as with navigating financial or logistical barriers to care.

Communication among team members is essential. Regular interdisciplinary rounds and case conferences facilitate coordinated decision-making, consistent patient messaging, and early intervention when complications or setbacks arise.

8.2 Early rehabilitation and prevention of contractures

Rehabilitation begins the moment the burn wound is closed. Early initiation of physiotherapy – often within days of epithelialization or grafting – is critical to maintaining mobility and preventing soft-tissue shortening.

Positioning and splinting counteract the natural tendency of healing tissues to contract. Splints are designed to hold joints in an antideformity position, typically at maximum extension or abduction, depending on the anatomical site. Splints may be static to maintain stretch during rest or dynamic to allow controlled motion during functional activities.

Daily range-of-motion exercises and passive stretching are vital components of rehabilitation. Stretching realigns collagen fibers along lines of tension, minimizing stiffness and promoting balanced remodeling. Therapists tailor exercise intensity to the patient's tolerance and stage of healing, with gradual progression to resistive strengthening once grafts have stabilized.

As part of the rehabilitative process, pressure garments and silicone sheeting are applied to mitigate hypertrophic scarring. These modalities, when used consistently, reduce capillary proliferation and collagen deposition, thereby improving scar texture and pliability. Compliance is enhanced through customized fitting, patient education, and regular follow-up for adjustments.

8.3 Functional rehabilitation and occupational therapy

The goal of functional rehabilitation is to restore maximal independence and reintegration into daily life. Occupational therapists play a central role by focusing on fine motor skills, adaptive equipment, and task-specific training.

In upper extremity burns, therapy emphasizes hand dexterity, grip strength, and coordination. Adaptive splints and assistive devices facilitate activities of daily living during recovery. For lower extremity burns, gait training and endurance exercises help restore mobility. Therapists also provide workplace and school reintegration plans, ensuring that patients can safely resume meaningful roles while continuing to protect healing skin.

8.4 Psychological and social rehabilitation

Burn scars are not merely physical – they carry deep psychological and social significance. Survivors often experience anxiety, depression, posttraumatic stress disorder (PTSD), and body image dissatisfaction, all of which can impede recovery and reintegration.

Early psychological intervention is essential. Cognitive behavioral therapy, mindfulness-based stress reduction, and peer support programs have demonstrated measurable improvements in coping and overall quality of life [93–95]. Group therapy allows patients to share experiences, fostering resilience and reducing isolation. In children, play therapy and family counseling address developmental and emotional needs associated with visible scarring.

Return to school, employment, and social activities is a critical milestone in recovery. Social workers help coordinate vocational rehabilitation, community reintegration programs, and cosmetic support services, such as specialized makeup or prosthetics. Advocacy for inclusive education and workplace accommodations remains an important component of comprehensive burn care.

8.5 Long-term scar surveillance and secondary interventions

Burn scars evolve over months to years, necessitating long-term follow-up to monitor maturation, contracture development, and psychosocial adaptation. Periodic evaluation using objective tools such as the VSS and POSAS provides standardized metrics for scar progression and response to therapy. Regular reassessment supports timely modification of garments, splints, or exercise regimens, preventing regression of earlier progress.

8.6 Education and patient empowerment

Patient and caregiver education forms the foundation of sustained recovery. Patients should understand the purpose of each therapy, the importance of adherence, and the long-term nature of scar maturation. Education also encompasses skin care, sun protection, hydration, and recognition of warning signs for ulceration or infection.

Empowering patients with knowledge promotes self-efficacy and compliance, both of which directly correlate with improved outcomes. Many burn centers employ dedicated education programs or discharge checklists to ensure consistent messaging and continuity of care.

8.7 Multidisciplinary models of care

Several leading burn centers worldwide have developed integrated scar management clinics, where surgeons, therapists, and psychologists collaboratively evaluate patients in a single visit. This model facilitates real-time treatment planning, minimizes fragmented care, and enhances patient satisfaction.

Emerging technologies – including telemedicine, virtual rehabilitation platforms, and mobile applications – now enable remote monitoring of exercise compliance and scar evolution. These innovations extend the reach of multidisciplinary care to patients in remote or resource-limited settings, promoting equitable access to long-term follow-up.

9. Future directions and conclusion

The field of burn scar management continues to evolve rapidly, propelled by advances in cell biology, biomaterials, and technology. Future strategies are increasingly focused on the prevention of fibrosis rather than its correction and on true tissue regeneration rather than replacement.

Emerging research into genomic and proteomic profiling of burn scars is uncovering molecular signatures that predict hypertrophic or keloid tendencies, paving the way for personalized antifibrotic therapies. Novel pharmacologic agents targeting TGF-β, CTGF, and mechanotransduction pathways hold promise in modulating scar formation at the molecular level.

Technological innovations such as 3D bioprinting, engineered dermal scaffolds, and exosome-based therapeutics are redefining reconstructive possibilities, allowing for patient-specific tissue constructs that integrate seamlessly with native skin. The integration of artificial intelligence (AI) and machine learning into scar assessment may soon enable automated quantification of scar morphology, vascularity, and maturation, providing objective metrics to guide treatment.

Furthermore, the incorporation of virtual reality (VR) and telerehabilitation platforms is enhancing access to physiotherapy, psychological counseling, and patient education – particularly for survivors in low-resource or remote settings. Global collaboration and capacity-building initiatives will be essential to ensure that these innovations are equitably translated into clinical practice worldwide.

Comprehensive burn scar management represents a synthesis of science, surgery, and compassion. Through an integrated framework encompassing prevention, conservative therapy, surgical reconstruction, regenerative medicine, and psychosocial rehabilitation, clinicians can restore both form and function while supporting the emotional recovery of burn survivors.

Advances in regenerative biology and technology are steadily transforming the outlook for patients, shifting scar care from mere mitigation toward functional and aesthetic restoration. Yet, the human element remains central: successful outcomes depend on multidisciplinary collaboration, long-term follow-up, and patient-centered care.

Ultimately, the management of burn scars is not only a technical pursuit but also a profoundly human one – dedicated to restoring identity, confidence, and quality of life to those who have endured devastating injuries.

Acknowledgments

The authors acknowledge using AI software for language editing in the chapter.

Author details

Chandler Hinson[1]*, Kimberly A. Donnellan[3], Andrew C. Bright[2] and Kevin Slaughter[2]

1 Frederick P. Whiddon College of Medicine, University of South Alabama, Mobile, USA

2 Division of Trauma, Acute Care Surgery, and Burns; USA Health, Mobile, USA

3 Skin and Laser Center; USA Health, Mobile, USA

*Address all correspondence to: chinson95@gmail.com

References

[1] Understanding Burns [Internet]. 2025. Available from: https://worldburn.org/understanding_burns.aspx. [Accessed: 2025-November-17]

[2] Rybarczyk MM, Schafer JM, Elm CM, Sarvepalli S, Vaswani PA, Balhara KS, et al. A systematic review of burn injuries in low- and middle-income countries: Epidemiology in the WHO-defined African Region. African Journal of Emergency Medicine. 2017;**7**:30–37

[3] Yakupu A, Zhang J, Dong W, Song F, Dong J, Lu S. The epidemiological characteristic and trends of burns globally. BMC Public Health. 2022;**22**:1596. DOI: 10.1186/s12889-022-13887-2

[4] Hu Y, Zhi L, Wang Y, Xiong F, Yu L, Hu X, et al. Global, regional, and national burden of burns from 1990 to 2021: A systematic analysis of prevalence, incidence, mortality, and disability-adjusted life years with projections to 2036. Journal of Craniofacial Surgery. 2025. DOI: 10.1097/SCS.0000000000011971

[5] Faour S, Farahat M, Aijaz A, Jeschke MG. Fibrosis in burns: An overview of mechanisms and therapies. American Journal of Physiology-Cell Physiology. 2023;**325**: C1545–57. DOI: 10.1152/ajpcell.00254.2023

[6] Korkmaz HI, Flokstra G, Waasdorp M, Pijpe A, Papendorp SG, de Jong E, et al. The complexity of the post-burn immune response: An overview of the associated local and systemic complications. Cells. 2023;**12**:345

[7] Finnson KW, McLean S, Di Guglielmo GM, Philip A. Dynamics of transforming growth factor beta signaling in wound healing and scarring. Advances in Wound Care. 2013;**2**:195–214. DOI: 10.1089/wound.2013.0429

[8] Tomasek JJ, Gabbiani G, Hinz B, Chaponnier C, Brown RA. Myofibroblasts and mechano-regulation of connective tissue remodelling. Nature Reviews Molecular Cell Biology. 2002;**3**:349–363. DOI: 10.1038/nrm809

[9] Pakshir P, Noskovicova N, Lodyga M, Son DO, Schuster R, Goodwin A, et al. The myofibroblast at a glance. Journal of Cell Science. 2020;**133**:jcs227900

[10] Schuster R, Younesi F, Ezzo M, Hinz B. The role of myofibroblasts in physiological and pathological tissue repair. Cold Spring Harbor Perspectives in Biology. 2023;**15**:a041231. DOI: 10.1101/cshperspect.a041231

[11] Kandhwal M, Behl T, Singh S, Sharma N, Arora S, Bhatia S, et al. Role of matrix metalloproteinase in wound healing. American Journal of Translational Research. 2022;**14**: 4391–4405

[12] Gauglitz GG, Korting HC, Pavicic T, Ruzicka T, Jeschke MG. Hypertrophic Scarring and Keloids: Pathomechanisms and Current and Emerging Treatment Strategies. Molecular Medicine. 2011;**17**:113–125. DOI: 10.2119/molmed.2009.00153

[13] Chiang RS, Borovikova AA, King K, Banyard DA, Lalezari S, Toranto JD, et al. Current concepts related to hypertrophic scarring in burn

injuries. Wound Repair and Regeneration. 2016;**24**:466–477

[14] Marshall CD, Hu MS, Leavitt T, Barnes LA, Lorenz HP, Longaker MT. Cutaneous scarring: basic science, current treatments, and future directions. Advances in Wound Care. 2018;**7**:29–45. DOI: 10.1089/wound.2016.0696

[15] Hong WX, Hu MS, Esquivel M, Liang GY, Rennert RC, McArdle A, et al. The role of hypoxia-inducible factor in wound healing. Advances in Wound Care. 2014;**3**:390–399

[16] Ruthenborg RJ, Ban -J-J, Wazir A, Takeda N, Kim J. Regulation of wound healing and fibrosis by hypoxia and hypoxia-inducible factor-1. Molecules and Cells. 2014;**37**:637–643. DOI: 10.14348/molcells.2014.0150

[17] L VDW, Varney S, Tomasek JJ. Mechanoregulation of the myofibroblast in wound contraction, scarring, and fibrosis: Opportunities for new therapeutic intervention. Advances in Wound Care. 2013;**2**:122–141. DOI: 10.1089/wound.2012.0393

[18] Hochman B, Tucci-Viegas VM, Monteiro PKP, França JP, Gaiba S, Ferreira LM. The action of CGRP and SP on cultured skin fibroblasts. Cent.eur.j. biol. 2014;**9**:717–726. DOI: 10.2478/s11535-014-0301-6

[19] Schäffer M, Beiter T, Becker HD, Hunt TK. Neuropeptides: Mediators of inflammation and tissue repair? Archives of Surgery. 1998;**133**: 1107–1116. DOI: 10.1001/archsurg.133.10.1107

[20] Kokubo K, Onodera A, Kiuchi M, Tsuji K, Hirahara K, Nakayama T. Conventional and pathogenic Th2 cells in inflammation, tissue repair, and fibrosis. Frontiers in Immunology. 2022;**13**:945063. DOI: 10.3389/fimmu.2022.945063

[21] Shirakami E, Yamakawa S, Hayashida K. Strategies to prevent hypertrophic scar formation: A review of therapeutic interventions based on molecular evidence. Burns & Trauma. 2020;**8**:tkz003. DOI: 10.1093/burnst/tkz003

[22] Mony MP, Harmon KA, Hess R, Dorafshar AH, Shafikhani SH. An Updated Review of Hypertrophic Scarring. Cells. 2023;**12**:678. DOI: 10.3390/cells12050678

[23] Butzelaar L, Ulrich MMW, Mink van der Molen AB, Niessen FB, Beelen RHJ. Currently known risk factors for hypertrophic skin scarring: A review. Journal of Plastic, Reconstructive & Aesthetic Surgery. 2016;**69**:163–169. DOI: 10.1016/j.bjps.2015.11.015

[24] Kim HJ, Kim YH. Comprehensive insights into keloid pathogenesis and advanced therapeutic strategies. International Journal of Molecular Sciences. 2024;**25**:8776. DOI: 10.3390/ijms25168776

[25] Jiao H, Zhang T, Fan J, Xiao R. The superficial dermis may initiate keloid formation: Histological analysis of the keloid dermis at different depths. Frontiers in Physiology. 2017;**8**:8. DOI: 10.3389/fphys.2017.00885

[26] Reinholz M, Guertler A, Schwaiger H, Poetschke J, Gauglitz GG. Treatment of keloids using 5-fluorouracil in combination with crystalline triamcinolone acetonide suspension: Evaluating therapeutic effects by using non-invasive objective

measures. Journal of the European Academy of Dermatology and Venereology. 2020;**34**:2436–2444. DOI: 10.1111/jdv.16354

[27] Walsh LA, Wu E, Pontes D, Kwan KR, Poondru S, Miller CH, et al. Keloid treatments: An evidence-based systematic review of recent advances. Systematic Reviews. 2023;**12**:42

[28] Berry CE, Downer M, Morgan AG, Griffin M, Liang NE, Kameni L, et al. The effects of mechanical force on fibroblast behavior in cutaneous injury. Frontiers in Surgery. 2023;**10**:1167067. DOI: 10.3389/fsurg.2023.1167067

[29] Phillips WA. Musculoskeletal issues in pediatric burn patients. Seminars in Plastic Surgery. 2024;**38**:154–156. DOI: 10.1055/s-0044-1782651

[30] den Kerckhove EV, Anthonissen M. Compression therapy and conservative strategies in scar management after burn injury. In: Téot L, Mustoe TA, Middelkoop E, Gauglitz GG, editors. Textbook on Scar Management: State of the Art Management and Emerging Technologies. Cham (CH): Springer; 2020. p. 227–231. https://www.ncbi.nlm.nih.gov/books/NBK586113/

[31] Edger-Lacoursière Z, Zhu M, Jean S, Marois-Pagé E, Nedelec B. Evidence supporting conservative scar management interventions following burn injury: A review article. Journal of Burn Care & Research. 2025;**46**:504–514. DOI: 10.1093/jbcr/irae204

[32] Ai J-W, Liu J, Pei S-D, Liu Y, Li D-S, Lin H, et al. The effectiveness of pressure therapy (15–25 mmHg) for hypertrophic burn scars: A systematic review and meta-analysis. Scientific Reports. 2017;**7**:40185

[33] Atiyeh BS, El Khatib AM, Dibo SA. Pressure garment therapy (PGT) of burn scars: Evidence-based efficacy. Annals of Burns and Fire Disasters. 2013;**26**:205–212

[34] Wiseman J, Ware RS, Simons M, McPhail S, Kimble R, Dotta A, et al. Effectiveness of Topical Silicone Gel and Pressure Garment Therapy for Burn Scar Prevention and Management in Children: A Randomized Controlled Trial. Vol. **34**. London, United Kingdom: SAGE Publications Ltd STM; 2020. p. 120–131. DOI: 10.1177/0269215519877516

[35] Rabello FB, Souza CD, Júnior JAF. Update on Hypertrophic Scar Treatment. Clinics (Sao Paulo). Vol. **69**. São Paulo, Brazil: Elsevier; 2014. p. 565–573. DOI: 10.6061/clinics/2014(08)11

[36] O'Brien L, Jones DJ. Silicone gel sheeting for preventing and treating hypertrophic and keloid scars. The Cochrane Database of Systematic Reviews. 2013;**2013**:CD003826. DOI: 10.1002/14651858.CD003826.pub3

[37] Gallant-Behm CL, Mustoe TA. Occlusion regulates epidermal cytokine production and inhibits scar formation. Wound Repair and Regeneration. 2010;**18**:235–244. DOI: 10.1111/j.1524-475x.2010.00575.x

[38] Mustoe TA. Silicone Gel for Scar Prevention. In: Téot L, Mustoe TA, Middelkoop E, Gauglitz GG, editors. Textbook on Scar Management: State of the Art Management and Emerging Technologies. Cham (CH): Springer; 2020. p. 203–208. https://www.ncbi.nlm.nih.gov/books/NBK586090/

[39] Bleasdale B, Finnegan S, Murray K, Kelly S, Percival SL. The use of silicone

adhesives for scar reduction. Advances in Wound Care. 2015;**4**:422–430. DOI: 10.1089/wound.2015.0625

[40] Jiang Q, Chen J, Tian F, Liu Z. Silicone gel sheeting for treating hypertrophic scars. Cochrane Database of Systematic Reviews. 2021;**2021**. DOI: 10.1002/14651858.CD013357.pub2

[41] Deflorin C, Hohenauer E, Stoop R, van Daele U, Clijsen R, Taeymans J. Physical management of scar tissue: A systematic review and meta-analysis. The Journal of Alternative and Complementary Medicine. 2020;**26**:854–865. DOI: 10.1089/acm.2020.0109

[42] Hosseini M, Brown J, Khosrotehrani K, Bayat A, Shafiee A. Skin biomechanics: A potential therapeutic intervention target to reduce scarring. Burns & Trauma. 2022;**10**:tkac036. DOI: 10.1093/burnst/tkac036

[43] Lin TR, Chou F-H, Wang -H-H, Wang R-H. Effects of scar massage on burn scars: A systematic review and meta-analysis. Journal of Clinical Nursing. 2023;**32**:3144–3154. DOI: 10.1111/jocn.16420

[44] Perera A, Perera C, Karunanayake A. Effectiveness of early stretching exercises for the quality of recovery of the upper limb in burnt patients. Physiotherapy. 2015;**101**: e1194. DOI: 10.1016/j.physio.2015.03.2119

[45] Lee J, Kim J. Minimal-invasive technologies for treatment of HTS and keloids: corticosteroids. In Téot L, Mustoe TA, Middelkoop E, Gauglitz GG, editors. Textbook on Scar Management: State of the Art Management and Emerging Technologies. Cham (CH): Springer; 2020. p. 243–250. https://www.ncbi.nlm.nih.gov/books/NBK586094/

[46] Sheng M, Chen Y, Li H, Zhang Y, Zhang Z. The application of corticosteroids for pathological scar prevention and treatment: Current review and update. Burns & Trauma. 2023;**11**:tkad009. DOI: 10.1093/burnst/tkad009

[47] Grigoryan KV, Kampp JT. Summary and evidence grading of over-the-counter scar treatments. International Journal of Dermatology. 2020;**59**:1136–1143. DOI: 10.1111/ijd.15060

[48] Ocampo-Candiani J, Vázquez-Martínez OT, Iglesias Benavides JL, Buske K, Lehn A, Acker C. The prophylactic use of a topical scar gel containing extract of Allium cepae, allantoin, and heparin improves symptoms and appearance of cesarean-section scars compared with untreated scars. Journal of Drugs in Dermatology. 2014;**13**:176–182

[49] Klifto KM, Asif M, Hultman CS. Laser management of hypertrophic burn scars: A comprehensive review. Burns & Trauma. 2020;**8**:tkz002. DOI: 10.1093/burnst/tkz002

[50] Kuo Y-R, Jeng S-F, Wang F-S, Chen T-H, Huang H-C, Chang P-R, et al. Flashlamp pulsed dye laser (PDL) suppression of keloid proliferation through down-regulation of TGF-β1 expression and extracellular matrix expression. Lasers in Surgery and Medicine. 2004;**34**:104–108

[51] Brewin MP, Docherty S, Heaslip V, Rhodes S, Ukoumunne OC, Burnett-Fry NC, et al. Early Laser for Burn Scars (ELABS) – Randomised controlled trial

of pulsed dye laser treatment and standard care versus standard care alone for the treatment of hypertrophic burn scars. Burns. 2025;**51**:107500. DOI: 10.1016/j.burns.2025.107500

[52] Li P, Zhang Q, Tao C, Liang H, Li D. Pulsed dye laser, fractional CO_2 laser, or combination for burn scar treatment: A systematic review. Lasers in Medical Science. 2025;**40**:389. DOI: 10.1007/s10103-025-04629-y

[53] Cai Y, Zeng X, Ying J, Zhu Y, Qiu Y, Xiang W. Efficacy and safety of pulsed dye laser for the treatment of surgical scars: A systematic review and meta-analysis. Lasers in Medical Science. 2022;**37**:1273–1282. DOI: 10.1007/s10103-021-03385-z

[54] Douglas H, Lynch J, Harms K-A, Krop T, Kunath L, van Vreeswijk C, et al. Carbon dioxide laser treatment in burn-related scarring: A prospective randomised controlled trial. Journal of Plastic, Reconstructive & Aesthetic Surgery. 2019;**72**:863–870

[55] Mahar PD, Spinks AB, Cleland H, Bekhor P, Waibel JS, Lo C, et al. Improvement of burn scars treated with fractional ablative CO_2 Lasers-A systematic review and meta-analysis using the Vancouver scar scale. Journal of Burn Care & Research. 2021;**42**:200–206

[56] Donnellan KA, Hinson CS, Blevins AC, Weaver KL, Lintner AC, Butts CC, et al. Treatment of chronic hypertrophic burn scars with a fractional CO_2 laser is well tolerated in an outpatient clinic setting. Annals of Plastic Surgery. 2023;**90**:444–446

[57] Peprah K, McCormack S. Fractionated CO_2 Laser for Scar Improvement: A Review of Clinical Effectiveness and Cost-Effectiveness [Internet]. Ottawa (ON): Canadian Agency for Drugs and Technologies in Health; 2019. Available from: https://www.ncbi.nlm.nih.gov/books/NBK546018/ [Accessed: 2025-November-14]

[58] Nisticò SP, Cannarozzo G, Campolmi P, Dragoni F, Moretti S, Patruno C, et al. Erbium laser for skin surgery: A single-center twenty-five years' experience. Medicines (Basel, Switzerland). 2021;**8**:74

[59] Kuehlmann B, Stern-Buchbinder Z, Wan DC, Friedstat JS, Gurtner GC. Beneath the surface: A review of laser remodeling of hypertrophic scars and burns. Advances in Wound Care. 2019;**8**:168–176. DOI: 10.1089/wound.2018.0857

[60] Meghe SR, Khan A, Jangid SD, Sarda B, Vangala N, Saoji V. Shedding light on acne scars: A comprehensive review of CO_2 vs. Erbium-Doped Yttrium Aluminium Garnet (Er:YAG) laser therapy. Cureus. 2024;**16**:e57572. DOI: 10.7759/cureus.57572

[61] Kim SG, Kim EY, Kim YJ, Lee SI. The efficacy and safety of ablative fractional resurfacing using a 2,940-Nm Er:YAG laser for traumatic scars in the early posttraumatic period. Archives of Plastic Surgery. 2012;**39**:232–237. DOI: 10.5999/aps.2012.39.3.232

[62] Alexiades-Armenakas MR, Dover JS, Arndt KA. The spectrum of laser skin resurfacing: Nonablative, fractional, and ablative laser resurfacing. Journal of the American Academy of Dermatology. 2008;**58**: 719–37. DOI: 10.1016/j.jaad.2008.01.003

[63] Kim KH, Geronemus RG. Nonablative Laser and Light Therapies for Skin Rejuvenation. Archives of Facial Plastic Surgery. Vol. **6**. Chicago, IL: SAGE Publications; 2004. p. 398–409. DOI: 10.1001/archfaci.6.6.398

[64] Waibel J, Wulkan AJ, Lupo M, Beer K, Anderson RR. Treatment of burn scars with the 1,550 nm nonablative fractional Erbium Laser. Lasers in Surgery and Medicine. 2012;**44**:441–446. DOI: 10.1002/lsm.22038

[65] Kang BY, Ibrahim SA, Weil A, Reynolds KA, Johnson T, Wilson S, et al. Treatment of surgical scars with combination pulsed dye and fractional nonablative laser: A randomized controlled trial. Annals of Surgery. 2022;**276**:975–980

[66] Ogawa R. Long-Pulsed 1064 nm Nd:YAG Laser Treatment for Keloids and Hypertrophic Scars. In Téot L, Mustoe TA, Middelkoop E, Gauglitz GG, editors. Textbook on Scar Management: State of the Art Management and Emerging Technologies [Internet]. Cham (CH): Springer; 2020. p. 271–278. https://www.ncbi.nlm.nih.gov/books/NBK586129/

[67] Thanh LTV, Quan TS, Anh LV, Hung TQ, Vuong NL. The efficacy of intense pulsed light in the treatment of keloids and hypertrophic scars. Journal of Lasers in Medical Sciences. 2023;**14**:e13. DOI: 10.34172/jlms.2023.13

[68] Corrêa FB, Castro JCD, Almeida IR, Farina-Junior JA, Coltro PS. Evaluation of contraction of the split-thickness skin graft using three dermal matrices in the treatment of burn contractures: A randomised clinical trial. Wound Repair and Regeneration. 2022;**30**:222–231. DOI: 10.1111/wrr.13002

[69] Aleman Paredes K, Selaya Rojas JC, Flores Valdés JR, Castillo JL, Montelongo Quevedo M, Mijangos Delgado FJ, et al. A comparative analysis of the outcomes of various graft types in burn reconstruction over the past 24 years: A systematic review. Cureus. 2024;**16**:e54277

[70] Balumuka DD, Galiwango GW, Alenyo R. Recurrence of post burn contractures of the elbow and shoulder joints: Experience from a Ugandan Hospital. BMC Surgery. 2015;**15**:103. DOI: 10.1186/s12893-015-0089-y

[71] Issa M, Badawi M, Bisheet G, Makram M, Elgadi A, Abdelaziz A, et al. Skin graft versus local flaps in management of post-burn elbow contracture. Cureus. 2021;**13**:e20768

[72] Ferland-Caron G, Kwan PO, Tredget EE. Free tissue transfer in the reconstruction of neck contractures after burn injury: A case series. European Burn Journal. 2023;**4**:248–258. DOI: 10.3390/ebj4020022

[73] Ma Z, Mo R, Chen C, Meng X, Tan Q. Surgical treatment of joint burn scar contracture: A 10-year single-center experience with long-term outcome evaluation. Annals of Translational Medicine. 2021;**9**:303–303. DOI: 10.21037/atm-20-4947

[74] Teufelsbauer M, Stickler S, Hammond DC, Hamilton G. Vascular endothelial growth factor expression of adipose-derived stromal cells and adipocytes initiated from fat aspirations. Aesthetic Plastic Surgery. 2025;**49**:4685–4695. DOI: 10.1007/s00266-024-04587-w

[75] Gan F, Liu L, Zhou Q, Huang W, Huang X, Zhao X. Effects of adipose-derived stromal cells and endothelial progenitor cells on adipose transplant survival and angiogenesis. PLOS ONE. 2022;**17**:e0261498. DOI: 10.1371/journal.pone.0261498

[76] Frommer ML, Langridge BJ, Beedie A, Jasionowska S, Awad L, Denton CP, et al. Exploring anti-fibrotic effects of adipose-derived stem cells: Transcriptome analysis upon fibrotic, inflammatory, and hypoxic conditioning. Cells. 2024;**13**:693

[77] Klinger M, Caviggioli F, Klinger FM, Giannasi S, Bandi V, Banzatti B, et al. Autologous fat graft in scar treatment. Journal of Craniofacial Surgery. 2013;**24**:1610–1615

[78] Liu J, Wang J, Zhang Q, Lu F, Cai J. Clinical, histologic, and transcriptomic evaluation of sequential fat grafting for morphea: A nonrandomized controlled trial. JAMA Dermatology. 2024;**160**:425–433. DOI: 10.1001/jamadermatol.2023.5908

[79] Wang M, Xu X, Lei X, Tan J, Xie H. Mesenchymal stem cell-based therapy for burn wound healing. Burns & Trauma. 2021;**9**:tkab002. DOI: 10.1093/burnst/tkab002

[80] Fujiwara O, Prasai A, Perez-Bello D, El Ayadi A, Petrov IY, Esenaliev RO, et al. Adipose-derived stem cells improve grafted burn wound healing by promoting wound bed blood flow. Burns & Trauma. 2020;**8**:tkaa009

[81] Hocking AM, Gibran NS. Mesenchymal stem cells: Paracrine signaling and differentiation during cutaneous wound repair. Experimental Cell Research. 2010;**316**:2213–2219. DOI: 10.1016/j.yexcr.2010.05.009

[82] Shahrokhi S, Anna A, Jeschke MG. The use of dermal substitutes in burn surgery: Acute phase. Wound Repair and Regeneration. 2014;**22**. DOI: 10.1111/wrr.12119

[83] Shokrani H, Shokrani A, Sajadi SM, Seidi F, Mashhadzadeh AH, Rabiee N, et al. Cell-seeded biomaterial scaffolds: The urgent need for unanswered accelerated angiogenesis. International Journal of Nanomedicine. 2022;**17**: 1035–1068

[84] Tartarini D, Mele E. Adult stem cell therapies for wound healing: Biomaterials and computational models. Frontiers in Bioengineering and Biotechnology. 2015;**3**:206. DOI: 10.3389/fbioe.2015.00206

[85] Dompe C, Moncrieff L, Matys J, Grzech-Leśniak K, Kocherova I, Bryja A, et al. Photobiomodulation—Underlying mechanism and clinical applications. Journal of Clinical Medicine. 2020;**9**:1724

[86] Hamblin MR. Mechanisms and Mitochondrial Redox Signaling in Photobiomodulation. Photochemistry and Photobiology. 2018;**94**:199–212. DOI: 10.1111/php.12864

[87] Khan I, Rahman SU, Tang E, Engel K, Hall B, Kulkarni AB, et al. Accelerated burn wound healing with photobiomodulation therapy involves activation of endogenous latent TGF-β1. Scientific Reports. 2021;**11**:13371. DOI: 10.1038/s41598-021-92650-w

[88] Desmoulière A, Geinoz A, Gabbiani F, Gabbiani G. Transforming growth factor-beta 1 induces alpha-smooth muscle actin expression in granulation tissue myofibroblasts and in quiescent and growing cultured fibroblasts. The Journal of Cell Biology.

1993;**122**:103–111. DOI: 10.1083/jcb.122.1.103

[89] Taflinski L, Demir E, Kauczok J, Fuchs PC, Born M, Suschek CV, et al. Blue light inhibits transforming growth factor-β1-induced myofibroblast differentiation of human dermal fibroblasts. Experimental Dermatology. 2014;**23**:240–246

[90] Kim YH, Kim HK, Choi JW, Kim YC. Photobiomodulation therapy with an 830-nm light-emitting diode for the prevention of thyroidectomy scars: A randomized, double-blind, sham device-controlled clinical trial. Lasers in Medical Science. 2022;**37**:3583–3590. DOI: 10.1007/s10103-022-03637-6

[91] Oh IY, Kim BJ, Kim MN, Kim CW, Kim SE. Efficacy of light-emitting diode photomodulation in reducing erythema after fractional carbon dioxide laser resurfacing: A pilot study. Dermatologic Surgery. 2013;**39**:1171–1176. DOI: 10.1111/dsu.12213

[92] de Araújo Pereira Venceslau SC, Ferreira JLS, Barros RMF, de Morais RM, Dos Santos HH, de Oliveira VMA, et al. Effects of photobiomodulation on re-epithelialization of burn wound: Protocol for a randomized controlled trial. Trials. 2022;**23**:573

[93] Shokre ES, Mohammed SEM, Elhapashy HMM, Elsharkawy NB, Ramadan OME, Abdelaziz EM. The effectiveness of the psychosocial empowerment program in early adjustment among adult burn survivors. BMC Nursing. 2024;**23**:45. DOI: 10.1186/s12912-024-01700-x

[94] Al-Ghabeesh SH, Mahmoud MM. Mindfulness and its positive effect on quality of life among chronic burn survivors: A descriptive correlational study. Burns. 2022;**48**:1130–1138. DOI: 10.1016/j.burns.2021.09.022

[95] Fauerbach JA, Gehrke AK, Mason ST, Gould NF, Milner SM, Caffrey J. Cognitive behavioral treatment for acute posttrauma distress: A randomized, controlled proof-of-concept study among hospitalized adults with burns. Archives of Physical Medicine and Rehabilitation. 2020;**101**: S16–25. DOI: 10.1016/j.apmr.2018.11.027

Chapter 10

Cutaneous Sequelae After Burn Injury: Pruritus, Dyspigmentation and Malignancy—Mechanisms and Management

Tunahan İnan and Selda Pelin Kartal

Abstract

Burn injuries can result in life-threatening complications as well as morbid sequelae that significantly impair quality of life in the long term. Cutaneous sequelae are also among the causes of these long-term morbidities. Postburn pruritus is one of the most common and troublesome complications, arising from pruritogenic and neuropathic mechanisms. Although it is most prevalent at discharge, it can persist for years. Dyspigmentation, including postburn hypopigmentation and hyperpigmentation, which is particularly noticeable in darker skin phototypes, is another common complication that causes psychological distress. The lack of a standard treatment algorithm for postburn pruritus and dyspigmentation, despite consensus, remains another significant problem. Cutaneous malignancies, most commonly squamous cell carcinoma, can develop on wounds left to heal secondarily after burns. These cutaneous malignancies are called Marjolin's ulcers and are important because they have a poor prognosis. This section summarizes the current pathophysiology of postburn pruritus, dyspigmentation, and malignancies, providing an evidence-based, practical assessment and management framework covering topical/systemic treatments, procedural approaches, and rehabilitation.

Keywords: burn, pruritus, hyperpigmentation, hypopigmentation, carcinoma, therapeutics

1. Introduction

Although advances in burn care have improved survival rates, chronic changes associated with scar tissue in the postburn period can affect patients' daily functioning and psychosocial well-being. In this context, postburn pruritus should be considered not merely as "itching," but as a complex symptom cluster involving intertwined inflammatory and neurosensory processes. Similarly, postburn dyspigmentation, ranging from hypopigmentation to hyperpigmentation, produces more pronounced clinical outcomes, particularly in darker skin phototypes, creating a measurable burden on quality of life beyond cosmetic concerns. On the other hand, malignant transformation (Marjolin's ulcer), which can develop in long-term nonhealing wounds or chronic scar areas, is rare but requires high clinical awareness due to the possibility of delayed diagnosis and aggressive course. This section aims to discuss current treatment options and supportive rehabilitation approaches in a practical framework by addressing the three main sequelae in terms of mechanisms, clinical evaluation, and management.

2. Postburn pruritus

2.1 Epidemiology

Data on the epidemiology of postburn pruritus has become clearer in recent years, thanks to large cohort studies. In a study of 637 adult burn survivors, the prevalence of pruritus at discharge was reported to be 93%; a gradual decrease was observed during follow-up, with rates remaining at 86%, 83%, and 73% at 6, 12, and 24 months, respectively [1]. Similarly, in another study involving 430 pediatric cases, pruritus was reported in 93% of patients at the time of discharge. The pruritus rate decreased over time during follow-up, recorded at 87% at the six-month evaluation, 78% at the one-year follow-up, and 64% at the end of the second year [2]. Female gender, burn area size, deep injuries requiring excision and grafting, young age, dry skin type, hypertrophic scar development, number of surgical interventions, and posttraumatic stress symptoms observed in the second week after the burn have been reported as risk factors that may be associated with the development of postburn pruritus [3, 4].

2.2 Pathogenesis

In the pathogenesis of postburn pruritus, both pruritogenic (peripheral) and neuropathic (central) components play a role; however, the neuropathic component is thought to be more dominant due to the more pronounced symptom control achievable with neuromodulatory agents and the frequent occurrence of paresthetic complaints during the recovery period [5]. Normally, numerous pruritogenic molecules, such as histamine, serotonin, bradykinin, substance P, calcitonin gene-related peptide (CGRP), and nerve growth factor (NGF), play a role in the formation of peripheral pruritus. The peripheral transmission of the itching sensation occurs via C fibers. Receptors such as the H1 histamine receptor, substance P-related receptors, protease-activated receptor-2 (PAR-2), and transient receptor potential vanilloid-1 (TRPV1) are also located at the ends of these fibers. On the other hand, keratinocytes can play an active role in initiating and maintaining pruritus by releasing neuropeptides after tissue damage; in this respect, they are thought to act as "itch-sensing" units. As scratching deepens epidermal damage and increases keratinocyte activation, the release of pruritogenic mediators is reinforced, perpetuating the well-known clinical "itch-scratch-itch" vicious cycle [6]. Postburn inflammation affects epidermal and dermal inflammation through various neuropeptides released from nerves in the skin. In this context, mediators such as histamine, CGRP, and substance P are released from keratinocytes, and these are reported to be the main transduction mediators in C fibers. Histamine has been shown to have a direct effect on itching via histamine-1 (H1) receptors; an increase in mast cell numbers has been demonstrated in postburn hypertrophic scars, and itching increases as scar thickness increases. In deep dermal burns, the decrease in substance P fibers during the acute phase is consistent with the initial absence of itching, while the increase in these fibers in the second week has been associated with the onset of itching [7, 8].

Peripheral neuroimmune interactions are not limited to the histamine axis alone. It has been reported that keratinocytes increase cytokines such as interleukin-31 (IL-31), which can induce a pronounced itching response by stimulating other immune cells such as T cells and mast cells. Additionally, thymic stromal lymphopoietin (TSLP) is released following activation of TRPV1, TRPV3, or PAR2 in keratinocytes. TSLP is a mediator that indirectly contributes to itching. It has been shown that the expression of IL-31 and its related receptors via the TRPV3 channel is increased in burn scar epidermis compared to intact skin. It has been reported that stimulation of TRPV3 in epidermal keratinocytes isolated from itchy burn scars triggers TSLP production; furthermore, TRPV3 is also highly expressed in fibroblasts from burn scars [9, 10].

Increased levels of mediators such as NGF, Substance P, histamine, and bradykinin in the periphery can trigger central nervous system (CNS) sensitization in the spinal cord and upper centers by more easily activating unmyelinated C fibers. In chronic burn cases, the upregulation of spinal calcium channels accompanying the increase in NGF/Substance P levels enhances this sensitization, leading to amplified itch transmission. Thus, itch can become partially independent of peripheral stimuli, taking on a more "autonomous" course and becoming chronic. In the chronic phase, it has been suggested that neuronal damage exceeding a certain threshold may trigger maladaptive response patterns. Nerve damage associated with burn injury and/or the treatment process causes a decrease in or alteration of the quality of sensory input reaching the CNS from the periphery (deafferentation). This disruption, combined with the weakening of inhibitory circuits in the spinal cord, reduces the "braking" of itch transmission; inhibitory neuron degeneration, interneuron hypoactivity, and disinhibition in descending antinociceptive pathways create a suitable environment for neuropathic itch. Long-term sensory changes may also have repercussions at the brain level; the postburn period may lead to changes in functional topography and cortical reorganization in the primary somatosensory cortex, supporting an impaired/distorted representation of the skin's "mapping," which may contribute to the persistence of itching [5, 6].

2.3 Clinical features

In the literature, pruritus associated with burns is classified according to its duration, with itching lasting ≥6 months defined as "chronic" and itching lasting <6 months defined as "acute" [11]. Less itching is observed in the face and neck areas compared to the upper and lower extremities and the back. Postburn itching becomes more pronounced in most patients, especially during the afternoon and evening hours. Factors that can exacerbate itching include dry skin, exposure to warm or hot environments, contact with warm or hot water, physical exertion, sweating, and fatigue. Conversely, in some cases, sleep, cold water, or cooler environments have been reported to reduce itching [12, 13].

Postburn pruritus, especially when severe and prolonged, becomes a significant symptom with biological, psychological, and social consequences. Itching can reduce daily functioning and attention, disrupt sleep patterns, and consequently negatively affect wound healing, prolonging the rehabilitation process. In chronic cases, many daily activities such as work life, treatment compliance, diet, sexual function, and leisure activities can be significantly affected. Day-and-night persistent itching can increase physical and mental fatigue over time, deepening disappointment, irritability/anger, social withdrawal, and psychological distress; an increase in anxiety and depressive symptoms may be seen along with a decrease in self-esteem and self-care capacity. In more severe cases, hopelessness and suicidal thoughts have also been reported. On the other hand, the scratching behavior triggered by pruritus poses direct clinical risks in burn patients. The main risks include disruption of skin integrity, traumatization of newly formed tissue, damage to donor sites, and increased risk of infection. This situation may prolong the hospital stay; in grafted patients, damage to the graft may necessitate additional intervention or additional grafts [5, 11].

There is currently no standardized measurement tool specific to this patient group for assessing the severity and impact of pruritus after burns. Therefore, although the Visual Analog Scale (VAS) and Numerical Rating Scale (NRS) are most commonly used in practice, these scales primarily reflect the "intensity" dimension and thus capture the continuity, spread, and impact of itching on functionality to a limited extent. When a more comprehensive assessment is required, multidimensional scales can be used. The 5-D Itch Scale can show changes in follow-up by inquiring about duration, intensity, course over time, daily life limitations, and distribution; however, it has been reported that the total score may remain low in cases with limited burn areas. The Leuven Itch Scale comprehensively assesses itching based on frequency, duration, intensity, discomfort, consequences, and affected area, and has been found useful in populations with chronic pruritus [14]. The Itch Man Scale is a detailed and recently validated pruritus assessment tool developed for children who have survived burns [15].

2.4 Management

Treatment options for postburn pruritus range from simple supportive approaches to pharmacological agents and complementary/rehabilitative interventions. However, due to the heterogeneity of methods in the current literature, the limited number of studies and sample sizes, and differences in outcome measures, a universally accepted, standardized treatment algorithm for postburn pruritus has not yet been established [5, 14, 16].

The effect of lemon balm tea on postburn pruritus was evaluated in a randomized controlled trial. A total of 90 patients were enrolled in the study and randomly assigned to control and intervention groups. The intervention group received 100 ml of lemon balm tea orally twice daily for two weeks in addition to standard burn care; the control group received only standard treatment. Itch severity was recorded daily using the VAS, and weekly averages for weeks 1, 2, and 3 were calculated for analysis. In terms of the course of itching, itching severity in the intervention group increased from week 1 to week 2 but decreased significantly from week 2 to week 3 and was found to be lower in week 3 compared to week 1. In contrast, in the control group, itching intensity gradually increased from week 1 to week 3, and this increase was found to be statistically significant [17]. Doxepin is a tricyclic antidepressant that strongly blocks histamine receptors.

Topical doxepin can be used on epithelialized burn areas not exceeding 20% of the total body surface area (TBSA). In a randomized controlled trial comparing topical doxepin with oral antihistamines, topical doxepin was reported to be more effective than antihistamines in reducing postburn itching intensity [18]. In contrast, another study comparing topical doxepin with a placebo cream control reported that topical doxepin was ineffective for postburn itching [19].

The effect of topical silicone gel on itching was evaluated in a randomized, placebo-controlled, double-blind, within-subject comparative study involving 23 patients. In each patient, one of two separate scar areas was treated with silicone gel, and the other with placebo cream, and itching was monitored using the Patient and Observer Scar Assessment Scale (POSAS). Although repeated measures analysis failed to show an overall treatment effect throughout follow-up, separate analysis of time points revealed lower itching reports in scars treated with silicone gel compared to placebo at three and six months [20]. The effect of the topical angiotensin-converting enzyme (ACE) inhibitor enalapril was investigated in a single-center, prospective, randomized, controlled, double-blind study. In 30 patients with hypertrophic scars and itching following second- or third-degree burns, 1% enalapril ointment was applied to one of two symmetrical scars and placebo to the other for six months (within-subject). Patients recorded their itching on a daily scale of 0–4, and at the end of treatment, the mean itching score was reported to be significantly lower on the side treated with enalapril compared to placebo [21].

The efficacy of a cream containing beeswax and herbal oil was evaluated in a randomized controlled trial, comparing it with aqueous cream used in standard care. Itching severity and duration were monitored using the VAS in a total of 52 participants. Additional clinical outcomes, such as application frequency, time to recurrence of itching after application, and the need for antipruritic medication, were also analyzed. The cream containing beeswax and herbal oil reduced itching more effectively, delayed symptom recurrence, and reduced the need for antipruritic medication compared to standard care [22].

A study evaluating the pharmacological control of burn-related pruritus with antihistamines used a blinded, crossover design. Patients were randomly assigned to one of four different drug regimens over a 16-day follow-up period; each treatment period lasted 4 days, and the treatment sequence was arranged according to a Graeco-Latin square design. With this randomization scheme, each participant received both the cetirizine + cimetidine combination and the diphenhydramine + placebo combination during the study period and served as their own control. Changes in itch severity were measured using the Numeric Itch Scale (NIS). The results showed that the cetirizine/cimetidine combination provided a significant reduction in itching at one and six hours after the first dose and a moderate reduction at 12 hours compared to the diphenhydramine/placebo combination [23].

Gabapentin has demonstrated clinical benefit in the management of postburn pruritus at doses generally ranging from 5–10 mg/kg/day in pediatric patients and 300–900 mg/day in divided doses in adults [24, 25]. A randomized study of gabapentin evaluated a total of 60 patients (n = 20 in each arm) and compared gabapentin, cetirizine, and combination therapies. The reduction in itch intensity was approximately 95% in the gabapentin group and remained at approximately 52% in the cetirizine group, and the difference was found to be statistically significant. The improvement achieved with combination therapy was reported to be close to that of gabapentin monotherapy (approximately 94%). The onset of gabapentin's effect was faster compared to cetirizine, as observed from the mean VAS scores on day 3: a 74% reduction was seen in the gabapentin group on day 3, while a 32% reduction was seen in the cetirizine group, and the difference was found to be statistically significant. At the end of follow-up, it was reported that all patients receiving gabapentin (alone or in combination) had a VAS score of 0–1 by day 28; however, the number of patients reaching this level was limited among those receiving cetirizine monotherapy (3 out of 20 patients) [25].

A double-blind, randomized, placebo-controlled, four-arm study evaluated a total of 80 adults (n = 20 per arm): pregabalin, cetirizine + pheniramine maleate, pregabalin + antihistamine combination, and placebo (vitamin B complex) were compared. All groups received massage with coconut oil as part of standard care. It was reported that itch control was significantly superior in the arms containing pregabalin (pregabalin monotherapy or in combination with antihistamines), with a response rate reaching approximately 95% in these groups; significantly better results were obtained compared to the antihistamine combination or massage alone [26].

Ondansetron is a widely used 5-hydroxytryptamine type 3 (5-HT_3) receptor antagonist for the prevention of chemotherapy-induced nausea and vomiting. Since the sensation of itching is largely transmitted via C fibers, and this transmission may be influenced by serotonin, 5-HT_3 receptor blockade has been considered a potential target for pruritus. A randomized controlled trial reported that a single 4 mg dose of ondansetron was superior to 25 mg of diphenhydramine in relieving postburn pruritus [27].

Extracorporeal shock wave therapy (ESWT) has been proposed to contribute to the reduction of postburn pruritus by suppressing Substance P and CGRP-related neurogenic inflammation through selective reduction in unmyelinated nerve fibers and neuro modulatory effects similar to "hyperstimulation analgesia." Randomized, sham-controlled studies in patients with reepithelialized burn scars have reported significant improvements in itch scores with ESWT. In one study, 46 patients were randomized to ESWT (n = 23) or sham (n = 23) arms; pruritus was assessed using the NRS, 5D-Itch Scale, and Leuven Itch Scale, and a significant decrease was observed in all scales in the ESWT group compared to sham after the third session [28]. Similarly, in another randomized study of 45 patients, low-dose ESWT (n = 23) was compared to sham (n = 22); follow-up with NRS and the 12-item Pruritus Severity Scale (12-PSS) reported a significant decrease in itch scores in the low-dose ESWT arm [29].

In a study comparing pulse dye laser (PDL) application with laser-free control areas, changes in burn-related pruritus were monitored using VAS. Participants were divided into four subgroups: adult–new scar (n = 8), adult–old scar (n = 10), child–new scar (n = 5), and child–old scar (n = 15). In each patient, the scar tissue was randomly divided into "treatment" and "control" areas; a total of three PDL sessions were applied to the treatment areas at monthly intervals. At follow-up, a significant decrease in itching scores was observed in both the treatment and control areas in the first month (after a single session), and this improvement was reported to be maintained at 6 and 12 months. The improvement in itching was more pronounced in the laser-treated areas compared to the control areas; the difference between the two areas reached a statistically significant level in the 6-month and 12-month evaluations [30].

The effect of high-intensity laser therapy (HILT) on postburn pruritus and quality of life was evaluated in a randomized, placebo-controlled study conducted in adult patients. A total of 49 patients were divided into active HILT (n = 24) and placebo laser (n = 25) groups; both groups received three sessions per week for sixweeks. All patients received standard care consisting of cetirizine (10 mg twice daily + 10 mg before bedtime) and were advised to perform scar massage with coconut oil four times daily (five minutes per session). Itch severity was assessed using the Itch Severity Scale (ISS), and quality of life impact was assessed using the modified Dermatology Life Quality Index (DLQI) at baseline, at six weeks, and at 12 weeks follow-up. In the active HILT arm, ISS scores were lower than placebo both at the end of treatment and at week 12; the improvement in DLQI was also more pronounced and sustained at follow-up [31].

In a prospective, randomized controlled study involving 20 adult patients with burn-related scars, the control area was compared with the same scar segments treated with ablative fractional carbon dioxide laser (AFCO$_2$L). A total of three laser sessions were applied to the treatment segment at four to six week intervals, and standard scar care was provided to all areas. Results were evaluated using POSAS scores at baseline and six weeks after the final session; follow-up data up to three years were also reported. At six weeks, a significant improvement in patient-reported POSAS scores for itching was observed in the AFCO$_2$L-treated segment compared to the control segment, but no persistent difference between segments was observed in the long-term follow-up [32]. In a study conducted by Hettrick et al., transcutaneous electrical nerve stimulation (TENS) was compared with standard care, and changes in itching were monitored using VAS. It was reported that in participants with baseline itching severity VAS ≥5, TENS application resulted in a statistically significant decrease in the mean itching severity measured by VAS compared to standard care [33].

Botulinum toxin type A (BTX-A) and intralesional triamcinolone acetonide (TAC) are among the therapeutic options that can be used in the management of postburn pruritus. In a single-blind study involving 60 patients, the selected scar area in cases of postburn pruritus was divided into two equal parts; BTX-A was injected into one half and TAC into the other. At the end of the study, a more pronounced and clinically significant improvement in pruritus severity and scar thickness was observed in the area treated with BTX-A compared to TAC. As a possible mechanism, it has been reported that BTX-A may reduce the expression of pruritus-related targets such as NGF and TRPV1/TRPA1; furthermore, by inhibiting neuropeptide release and inflammation associated with neuropathic pruritus, it may enhance the efficacy and durability of the treatment response when added as an adjuvant to TAC [34]. The efficacy of massage in postburn pruritus has been examined in two randomized controlled trials comparing it with standard care. Both studies reported that massage application resulted in a statistically significant reduction in itch scores compared to standard care and could reduce the average itch intensity [35, 36].

3. Postburn dyspigmentation

3.1 Epidemiology

In the follow-up of burn survivors, pigmentation disorders were observed in 83.7% of cases; these could present as hyperpigmentation or depigmentation/

hypopigmentation [37]. A study conducted on the pediatric population reported that hypopigmentation could develop in 25% of cases after burns [38].

3.2 Pathogenesis

Postburn pigmentation patterns are largely related to the depth of the burn. Since first-degree burns are limited to the superficial layers of the epidermis, permanent color changes are generally not expected after reepithelialization. In contrast, depigmentation is more common in second- and third-degree burns because epidermal melanocytes and melanosomes are significantly damaged. Repigmentation (RP) in second-degree burns is achieved by the proliferation and migration of melanocytes at the wound edge and the migration of melanoblasts located in the surrounding skin or preserved hair follicle units, which differentiate into mature melanocytes. In third-degree burns, the "reserve" pool of melanocytes and melanoblasts decreases due to the destruction of dermal adnexa; regeneration relies more on (i) the proliferation and migration of melanocytes at the wound edge and (ii) the migration and differentiation of melanoblasts in the bulge region of the hair follicle at the wound edge [39]. The dynamic change in wound pH is an important microenvironmental factor affecting melanogenesis. It has been reported that wound pH can shift toward alkaline during the healing process, return to neutral with epithelialization, and remain higher in deep burns. Intramelanosomal pH is closely related to tyrosinase activity; more acidic melanosomal pH decreases tyrosinase activity, while pH closer to neutral can increase activity and contribute to skin color differences.

The inflammatory response can contribute to hyperpigmentation by reshaping the wound microenvironment in a way that supports melanocyte activation. During this process, mediators such as stem cell factor (SCF), basic fibroblast growth factor (bFGF), granulocyte-macrophage colony-stimulating factor (GM-CSF), monocyte chemoattractant protein-1 (MCP-1), prostaglandins, leukotrienes, thromboxanes, histamine, and carbon monoxide may increase. Prostaglandin E2 (PGE2) and F2α (PGF2α), leukotriene C4 (LTC4) and D4 (LTD4), and thromboxane B2 (TXB2) can increase tyrosinase activity and melanosome transport; histamine has been shown to stimulate melanogenesis, particularly via the H2 receptor. In contrast, Dickkopf 1 (DKK1), transforming growth factor-beta 1 (TGF-β1), and factors such as IL-1, IL-6, and tumor necrosis factor-alpha (TNF-α) may have inhibitory effects; the clinical pattern is thought to depend on the balance of stimulatory and inhibitory signals [39, 40]. Nitric oxide (NO) can enhance melanogenesis by increasing tyrosinase activity in melanocytes through upregulation via cyclic guanosine monophosphate (cGMP)-dependent pathways and microphthalmia-associated transcription factor (MITF). Elevated plasma nitrite/nitrate levels in burn patients have been associated with increased NO production after burns; the rapid release of NO in the early phase also supports this role [41].

3.3 Clinical features

Hyperpigmentation is more common in partial-thickness burns that heal without surgery; this is thought to be related to postburn inflammation stimulating melanocytes in intact epidermal structures, increasing their proliferation and elevating melanin accumulation in the lesion area. Skin grafting applied to partial-thickness and full-thickness burns may also be accompanied by hyperpigmentation due to the inflammation-induced increase in melanogenesis. Pigmentation irregularities during the healing process are expected to gradually fade, allowing the skin color to approach normal. In contrast, hypopigmentation is more pronounced and takes longer to resolve after full-thickness burns in dark-skinned patients. This is because full-thickness skin loss causes damage to melanocytes and melanocyte stem cells; the migration of melanocytes from the wound edge to the lesion area is also often impossible. Furthermore, the developing scar tissue further restricts melanocyte migration, reducing melanin production [42, 43].

3.4 Management

3.4.1 Hyperpigmentation treatment

A study evaluating 45 patients with postinflammatory hyperpigmentation (PIH), including cases of postburn pigmentation, compared salicylic acid, topical tretinoin, and a combination of these two agents. Combination therapy was found to be superior to both monotherapies in reducing hyperpigmentation; it was also associated with a low incidence of side effects, a low recurrence rate, and good tolerability [44]. The efficacy of a topical silicone film dressing in patients with superficial burns on the face and neck was compared with standard care, and silicone gel application was shown to be associated with a statistically significant reduction in the modified Vancouver Scar Scale (mVSS) pigmentation subscore [45]. In a series of 19 cases evaluating the efficacy of intense pulsed light (IPL) in the treatment of PIH after burns, more than 78% of patients showed more than 50% clinical improvement, and approximately 32% showed more than 75% improvement [46]. In another study, a total of 53 postburn PIH plaques were examined in 14 patients; the combined use of two IPL sessions and a modified Kligman formula (tretinoin, vitamin C, triamcinolone, and hydroquinone) provided a faster and stronger clinical response compared to the group treated with the modified Kligman formula alone for two months [47].

A study involving 35 patients with postburn PIH in the facial area evaluated the clinical outcomes of microplasma radiofrequency application. The series reported an improvement in hyperpigmentation of over 51% in 32 patients. Pain was highlighted as one of the main issues limiting the practical use of this method. The mean pain score, assessed by VAS, was 6.7 ± 0.7; it was stated that patients frequently complained of pain during treatment [48]. Erbium:YAG laser was used to evaluate a total of 96 postburn hyperpigmented scars in 24 patients; a marked improvement in hyperpigmentation was reported. Complete disappearance was reported in all lesions with a "black powder tattoo" appearance in the series, while clinical improvement was observed in approximately 93% of small dark macule/freckle-like lesions [49]. In a study involving eight patients with hyperpigmentation following deep second- or third-degree burns, approximately 80% improvement in dyschromia was achieved with fractional nonablative erbium laser [50]. A 2018 report described the successful treatment of two Fitzpatrick type III patients with burn scars using a combination of PDL and nonablative fractional laser; it also suggested that nonablative laser could be used in conjunction with fat micrografting [51]. In a larger case series with eight years of experience, fractional laser was combined with "micro-fat graft" injection in 288 patients with burn scars; it was reported to reduce hyperpigmentation, with overall improvement rates ranging from 40 to 80% and high patient satisfaction [52].

In 19 cases of postburn hyperpigmentation, mechanical dermabrasion was applied to the hyperpigmented areas using a diamond burr, followed by the preparation of a partial-thickness skin graft slightly larger than the defect and 0.12 inches thick, harvested from the plantar medial region using a pneumatic dermatome. The graft was then secured to the raw surface with simple sutures and/or compressive dressing. At the one-year follow-up, 15 patients reported being "very satisfied," and 4 patients reported being "relatively satisfied"; The mean appearance improvement score reached 4.5, and the VSS score decreased from 9.53 to 2.53 [53].

A 2023 review proposed a stepwise treatment algorithm for postburn hyperpigmentation. According to this, in cases of hyperpigmentation developing within the first 12 months after a burn, observation is preferred without initiating treatment until scar maturation is complete. After this period, topical agents, which are the least invasive options, are recommended in the first step: tyrosinase inhibitors (hydroquinone, 4-n-butylresorcinol) and, when necessary, combinations such as chemical peeling, tretinoin, corticosteroids, azelaic acid, kojic acid, arbutin, ascorbic acid, and soy extract. However, it should be noted that in some studies, the etiology of PIH is not clearly defined, and efficacy/safety data for hyperpigmentation directly related to burns are limited. In cases unresponsive to topical agents, PDL, Q-switched ruby laser, and nonablative fractional erbium/thulium lasers may be considered as second-line options; however, the level of evidence and optimal protocols remain unclear, and patient selection, parameters, and posttreatment care should be meticulously planned, considering that lasers may trigger PIH. In selected cases, particularly on the face, microplasma radiofrequency may be an alternative/adjuvant option; surgery, however, should be considered with more limited indications, particularly for hyperpigmentation developing in grafted areas, due to additional donor site morbidity [54].

3.4.2 Hypopigmentation treatment

If the size and location of the hypopigmented scar are appropriate, primary suturing after scar excision is the preferred option. When primary closure is not possible, the scar tissue is excised, and the groundwork for RP is then prepared. Dermabrasion, applied for this purpose, is based on the controlled removal of the epidermis down to the papillary dermis. Laser applications or microneedling methods can also be used for similar purposes. The goal during the RP phase is to restore melanocytes to the hypopigmented area prepared by dermabrasion and thus bring the color of the lesion as close as possible to the preburn or surrounding skin tone. Different surgical RP techniques can be applied for this purpose [55].

Full-thickness skin grafting (FTSG) for the treatment of pigmentation disorders involves obtaining the entire thickness of the epidermis and dermis, usually with the aid of a scalpel. Split-thickness skin grafting (STSG), on the other hand, involves only a portion of the epidermis and dermis. Both methods have been reported to be effective surgical techniques for treating hypopigmented scars resulting from burns [56, 57]. In the tiny epidermal particle graft (TEPG) technique, a thin skin graft is taken; it is passed through a skin expander several times and then cut into as small particles as possible with a cold knife. The resulting TEPG is evenly distributed over an oily gauze compress the size of the depigmented lesion. It allows for the treatment of an area three to five times larger than the donor site. In suction blister epidermal grafting (SBEG), epidermal blisters are created in normally pigmented donor skin using negative pressure; the blister roof is harvested as a graft and transferred to the depigmented area [58].

In a study involving 30 patients with burn-induced depigmentation, the cases were divided into two groups: Group I received TEPG, and Group II received SBEG. At 12 months postoperatively, the area of RP was quantitatively assessed using Image-Pro Plus; RP >75% was defined as an "optimal" response, and RP >90% as an "excellent" response. A significant difference in pigmentation was reported between the groups; optimal RP was achieved in 12 patients in Group I and 9 patients in Group II, while excellent RP was achieved in 14 patients in Group I and 10 patients in Group II. It was emphasized that both methods can provide high RP, but TEPG is less traumatic and has more predictable results compared to SBEG; therefore, it may be a preferable option, especially in large depigmented areas [59]. In the thin minigrafting technique (minipunch), small pockets are created in the recipient depigmented area at 4 mm intervals using a 0.25 mm minipunch, reaching partial thickness to the dermis. A very thin split-thickness skin graft is taken from the donor site using a Thiersch-type scalpel, divided into small pieces, and placed into the recipient sites, which are then immobilized with surgical tape for ~ 1 week. Its main advantage is that it can treat areas up to 25 times larger than the donor site [60].

Autologous melanocyte transplantation, applied together with keratinocytes and targeting melanocyte recolonization in depigmented areas, is an alternative or complementary approach to grafting. Cell suspensions, especially in extensive and deep burns, can allow treatment of larger areas with a donor-to-recipient ratio of approximately 1:10. For this purpose, a live autologous skin cell suspension is prepared intraoperatively in spray form using the ReNovaCell Autologous Cell Harvesting Device and applied to the wound bed. It has been reported that the combination of the noncultured autologous skin cell suspension (NCASCS) technique with nonablative microneedling in large (>10 cm^2) hypopigmented burn scars can support RP; furthermore, the addition of postoperative excimer laser can provide synergy by increasing melanocyte activation and migration [61, 62].

Although tissue engineering-based skin substitutes have been developed for wound coverage and tissue repair, hypopigmentation remains a significant limitation, as pigmentation mismatch is frequently reported in full-thickness skin substitutes. Therefore, current studies focus on melanocyte integration into skin substitutes, hair follicle-derived cells, and induced pluripotent stem cell (iPSC)-based strategies for more physiological melanin production and transfer in the long term. The ability to recreate "skin-like" tissues with preserved multilayered structure and more appropriate pigmentation, and to optimize these approaches to support postburn RP, holds promise for depigmentation treatment [63].

In recent years, device-based and adjuvant medical options for scar sequelae have increased; however, while the level of evidence for postburn hypopigmentation is limited, promising methods for permanent RP have been reported. Medical tattooing is a low-cost, noninvasive, and low-complication camouflage/RP option for postburn leukoderma, which can improve quality of life and social participation by reducing the appearance of color loss [64][. A review focusing on postburn hypopigmented scars summarized nonsurgical options under the headings of E-light (IPL + radiofrequency + cooling combination), laser-based approaches (especially fractional CO_2 laser), and laser-assisted drug delivery (LADD). Data suggest that LADD may enhance RP with agents such as bimatoprost, tretinoin, and pimecrolimus by increasing the penetration of topical agents through the microchannels created by the fractional laser [65]. Furthermore, nonsteroidal antiinflammatory drugs such as tacrolimus and targeted mediators such as melanocyte-stimulating hormones are expected to become more clinically relevant, especially when combined with laser-assisted topical delivery protocols. However, stronger clinical studies are needed regarding efficacy, durability, optimal protocols, and patient selection [65, 66].

4. Malignancy

4.1 Epidemiology

Although the concept of Marjolin's ulcer has historically been used to describe cutaneous malignancies developing on the basis of burn scar tissue, the current approach acknowledges that this condition is not limited to burns alone; chronic inflammation, chronic wounds/ulceration, and long-term tissue damage can also predispose to similar malignant transformation. However, the most frequently reported underlying cause in the etiology of cases remains burn scar tissue [67]. Determining the true incidence is difficult; however, the literature reports that the rate of Marjolin's ulcer development in deep burns left to secondary healing ranges from approximately 0.77 to 2.0%. In terms of histopathological distribution, squamous cell carcinoma (SCC) is by far the most common malignancy encountered in Marjolin's ulcers. In addition, rarer histological types such as basal cell carcinoma, melanoma, sarcomas, squamo-basal variants, dermatofibrosarcoma protuberans, and various mesenchymal tumors have also been described at the case report level. Marjolin's ulcers are most frequently seen in the fifth decade and are approximately 2:1 or 3:1 more common in men than in women; this difference is probably related to the higher incidence of burns in this group [68]. However, the latent period is inversely proportional to age at the time of injury: the latent interval is generally longer in childhood and tends to be shorter in older age [69].

4.2 Pathogenesis

Burn scars create a microenvironment characterized by prolonged tissue destruction and reepithelialization, increased proliferation, and the potential to act as a "mutagenic focus." Chronic inflammation enhances cellular division and growth factor release while suppressing apoptosis; accelerated transformation, particularly at the wound margin, facilitates the accumulation of mutations [70]. In addition, inadequate perfusion, relative avascularity, and lymphatic obliteration or obstruction may weaken "immune surveillance," increasing the potential for transformed cells to evade the immune system. Disruptions in adhesion molecules and increased growth factors are important in invasion and metastasis; growth factors can increase cellular motility via fibroblast-mediated epithelial–mesenchymal transition (EMT), and clinically, spread often occurs via the lymphatic route. Although the fibrous tissue surrounding the ulcer may initially form a barrier, it has been suggested that lymphatic spread may be facilitated after extensive surgical excision [71–73].

According to the "two-hit hypothesis," burn trauma initiates early mutations as the first "hit"; the second "hit" triggers malignant transformation. Individual predispositions, such as abnormalities in human leukocyte antigen (HLA) subtypes (HLA-DR4), p53 (TP53), and Fas receptor (FasR) pathways, may play a role in this process. The increased clinical risk is more pronounced in full-thickness burns left to secondary healing, nonhealing/easily ulcerating fragile scars, and scars exposed to high mechanical stress (crossing joint lines); UV and ionizing radiation may also facilitate the procarcinogenic "second hit" [68, 74, 75].

4.3 Clinical features

Marjolin ulcers are generally classified into two main groups based on clinical timing. Acute Marjolin ulcer is a relatively rare condition and is defined by the emergence of malignant transformation within the first year following injury. In contrast, chronic Marjolin ulcers are more common; malignancy developing after a latent period of more than 12 months following injury or scar formation corresponds to this group. The latent period in chronic ulcers can vary widely; the average latent period is thought to be approximately 30 years [76]. Although Marjolin ulcers can theoretically develop in any anatomical region, SCCs associated with Marjolin ulcers have been reported to develop more frequently in the lower extremities, where perfusion is relatively low and the risk of trauma is higher [77]. Any wound that develops on chronic scar tissue and does not heal or exhibits ulcerative features should raise suspicion of Marjolin's ulcer in the clinician. The most typical clinical appearance is an elevated or everted-edged ulcer with surrounding induration and a mostly flat base. The main findings that increase suspicion of malignancy in chronic wounds are exophytic growth, irregularity at the ulcer base, and the presence of excessive granulation tissue extending beyond the ulcer margin. In some cases, the lesion may present as an exophytic mass mimicking granulation tissue [76, 78].

4.4 Management

The diagnosis is confirmed by histopathological evaluation. Excisional biopsy is the gold standard for diagnosis; however, since it cannot always be performed, a 4–6 mm full-thickness incisional biopsy may also be sufficient. Bozkurt et al. proposed a sampling approach based on lesion size: biopsy from two different areas for tumors smaller than 2.5 cm, four biopsies for lesions between 2.5 and 5 cm, and six biopsies for lesions larger than 5 cm [79, 80]. After the diagnosis is confirmed by biopsy, patients should be evaluated according to standard oncological principles for staging purposes. Although there is no internationally accepted TNM system specific to Marjolin ulcers, it is known that these tumors can be more aggressive than classic cutaneous malignancies. A detailed regional lymph node examination must be performed during clinical evaluation; appropriate imaging should be planned for distant metastasis screening based on the clinical characteristics of the lesion and the patient's risk profile. For this purpose, chest X-ray, brain computed tomography (CT), and abdominal ultrasonography can be considered as basic methods; advanced cross-sectional imaging techniques such as CT or magnetic resonance imaging (MRI) can be used in necessary cases. The distant metastasis rate has been reported in the literature as 27.5%, while the recurrence rate has been reported to be between 20% and 50% [81, 82].

Prevention is likely the most effective strategy in the management of Marjolin ulcers. Leaving burn wounds to heal secondarily significantly increases the risk of Marjolin ulcer development in the long term. Therefore, reexcision may be considered for fragile, easily ulcerated, or repeatedly traumatized burn scars; at the very least, close clinical follow-up of these areas for malignant transformation is recommended. Treating deep burns in the acute phase with an appropriate surgical approach (excision and grafting) stands out as a protective measure that reduces the risk of Marjolin's ulcer developing in the future [68, 76]. Although there is no standardized treatment protocol for Marjolin's ulcers, the basic approach is surgical excision. While there is no complete consensus on the horizontal surgical margins for wide local excision of the primary tumor focus, a surgical margin of 2–4 cm is generally recommended. Intraoperative frozen-section examination can be used to confirm complete resection. There is also no clear consensus on the depth of excision. The choice of skin graft or flap for reconstruction is planned according to the location of the lesion; some studies prefer skin grafts because recurrence can be more easily monitored. Amputation may also be considered in selected cases based on the location, depth, extent, and functional requirements of the lesion [76, 78, 83]. Mohs surgery may be considered as an option in cosmetically sensitive areas or in cases of recurrence [76, 84].

The role of prophylactic lymph node dissection in regional lymph node management is controversial, and there is no clear consensus on this approach. In patients with clinically positive lymph nodes, biopsy and/or therapeutic lymph node dissection is recommended to confirm nodal involvement. Although studies have reported that prophylactic sentinel lymph node biopsy (SLNB) may be useful in the evaluation of regional lymph nodes in patients with Marjolin's ulcer, there is no consensus on the indication for prophylactic SLNB. Some authors state that SLNB may be considered in selected cases to detect micrometastases and improve staging, even if lymph nodes are negative on clinical examination [81, 85]. There is no standard consensus on neoadjuvant/adjuvant treatments for Marjolin's ulcer. However, chemoradiotherapy may be administered in selected cases for symptom control and palliative benefit in widespread metastatic disease. According to the recommendations of Özek et al., radiotherapy is indicated in cases with inoperable regional lymph node metastasis, in cases where positive lymph nodes are detected after nodal dissection and/or high-grade (grade 3) tumors are present, in cases where the tumor diameter is >10 cm with lymph node involvement, and in head and neck cases where nodal positivity is detected. Furthermore, even if lymph nodes are negative after nodal dissection, the indication for radiotherapy may be reconsidered in high-grade and large-diameter lesions [86].

Chemotherapy is generally considered in patients who are not candidates for surgery; reported regimens may include combinations of cisplatin, methotrexate, and bleomycin, as well as topical or systemic 5-fluorouracil (5-FU). In selected cases – particularly in disease located in the extremities – hyperthermic intraarterial limb perfusion is discussed as an alternative approach. Although immune checkpoint inhibitors have shown signs of efficacy in early-phase data for metastatic squamous cell Marjolin ulcer, stronger studies are needed to clarify their place in clinical practice; moreover, cost is a significant factor limiting their use [87].

5. Conclusion

Postburn cutaneous sequelae represent a significant area of morbidity that can affect patients' functionality and quality of life for a long time after the acute phase. Postburn pruritus should be considered a complex symptom that may involve peripheral pruritogenic processes along with significant neuropathic components; effective control should be targeted due to its consequences, such as sleep disturbance, decreased attention, and secondary tissue damage triggered by scratching. Dyspigmentation, on the other hand, is related to burn depth, preservation of melanocyte reserves, and the inflammatory microenvironment, and it can lead to a more pronounced clinical and psychosocial burden, especially in darker skin phototypes. Although treatment options are increasing, the heterogeneity of existing studies, which focus specifically on postburn pruritus and dyspigmentation, makes it difficult to develop a standard algorithm. Therefore, management should be planned within a practical and individualized framework, supported by procedural interventions and rehabilitation approaches in appropriate cases, using stepwise topical/systemic treatments. On the other hand, although Marjolin's ulcer, which can develop on the basis of chronic wounds or unstable scars, is rare, it requires regular clinical evaluation and a low biopsy threshold for suspicious lesions due to its potential for delayed diagnosis and aggressive course.

Author details

Tunahan İnan* and Selda Pelin Kartal
Department of Dermatology and Venereology, Ankara Etlik City Hospital, Ankara, Turkey

*Address all correspondence to: drtunainan@gmail.com

References

[1] Carrougher GJ, Martinez EM, McMullen KS, et al. Pruritus in adult burn survivors: Postburn prevalence and risk factors associated with increased intensity. Journal of Burn Care & Research 2013;**34**:94–101

[2] Schneider JC, Nadler DL, Herndon DN, et al. Pruritus in pediatric burn survivors: Defining the clinical course. Journal of Burn Care & Research. 2015;**36**(1):151–158. DOI: 10.1097/BCR.0000000000000145

[3] Van Loey NE, Bremer M, Faber AW, Middelkoop E, Nieuwenhuis MK. Itching following burns: Epidemiology and predictors. British Journal of Dermatology. 2008;**158**(1):95–100. DOI: 10.1111/j.1365-2133.2007.08278.x

[4] Sood RF, Hocking AM, Muffley LA, et al. Race and melanocortin 1 receptor polymorphism R163Q are associated with post-burn hypertrophic scarring: A prospective cohort study. Journal of Investigative Dermatology. 2015;**135**(10):2394–2401. DOI: 10.1038/jid.2015.197

[5] Chung BY, Kim HB, Jung MJ, et al. Post-burn pruritus. International Journal of Molecular Sciences. 2020;**21**(11):3880. DOI: 10.3390/ijms21113880

[6] Ahuja RB, Chatterjee P. Postburn pruritus: A practical review. Indian Journal of Burns. 2014;**22**(1):13–21

[7] Choi YH, Kim KM, Kim HO, Jang YC, Kwak IS. Clinical and histological correlation in post-burn hypertrophic scar for pain and itching sensation. Annals of Dermatology. 2013;**25**(4):428–433. DOI: 10.5021/ad.2013.25.4.428

[8] Kwak IS, Choi YH, Jang YC, Lee YK. Immunohistochemical analysis of neuropeptides (protein gene product 9.5, substance P, and calcitonin gene-related peptide) in hypertrophic burn scars with pain and itching. Burns. 2014;**40**(8):1661–1667. DOI: 10.1016/j.burns.2014.04.004

[9] Yang YS, Cho SI, Choi MG, Choi YH, Kwak IS, Park CW, Kim HO. Increased expression of three types of transient receptor potential channels (TRPA1, TRPV4 and TRPV3) in burn scars with post-burn pruritus. Acta Dermato-Venereologica. 2015;**95**:20–24. DOI: 10.2340/00015555-1858

[10] Lee MY, Shin E, Kim H, Kwak IS, Choi Y. Interleukin-31, interleukin-31RA, and OSMR expression levels in post-burn hypertrophic scars. Journal of Pathology and Translational Medicine. 2018;**52**:307–313. DOI: 10.4132/jptm.2018.08.03

[11] Aktas H, Tuncbilek Z, Hidiroğlu S. Evaluation of the effect of post-burn pruritus on patients' quality of life and experiences. Burns. 2026;**52**(1):107808. 107808. DOI: 10.1016/j.burns.2025.107808

[12] Gauffin E, Öster C, Gerdin B, Ekselius L. Prevalence and prediction of prolonged pruritus after severe burns. Journal of Burn Care & Research. 2015;**36**(3):405–413

[13] Parnell LK, Nedelec B, Rachelska G, LaSalle L. Assessment of pruritus characteristics and impact on burn survivors. Journal of Burn Care & Research. 2012;**33**(3):407–418

[14] Nedelec B, LaSalle L. Postburn itch: A review of the literature. Wounds. 2018;**30**(1):E118–E124

[15] Morris V, Murphy LM, Rosenberg M, Rosenberg L, Holzer 3rd CE, Meyer 3rd WJ. Itch assessment scale for the pediatric burn survivor. Journal of Burn Care & Research. 2012;**33**: 419–424

[16] Andrade LF, Abdi P, Kooner A, et al. Treatment of post-burn pruritus: A systematic review and meta-analysis. Burns. 2024;**50**(2):293–301. DOI: 10.1016/j.burns.2023.09.012

[17] Fayazi N, Rahzani K, Rezaei K, Alizadeh SA. The effect of complementary medicine-based intervention on burning patients' pruritus. International Journal of Pharmacy and Phytopharmacological Research. 2019;**9**(5):51–56

[18] Demling RH, DeSanti L. Topical doxepin significantly decreases itching and erythema in the chronically pruritic burn scar. Wounds. 2003;**15** (7):195–200

[19] Kwa KAA, Legemate CM, Pijpe A, et al. Doxepin cream is not effective in reducing itch in burn scar patients: A multicenter triple-blind randomized clinical crossover trial. Burns. 2020;**46** (2):340–346. DOI: 10.1016/j.burns.2019.11.006

[20] So K, Umraw N, Scott J, Campbell K, Musgrave M, Cartotto R. Effects of enhanced patient education on compliance with silicone gel sheeting and burn scar outcome: A randomized prospective study. Journal of Burn Care & Rehabilitation. 2003;**24**(6):411–420. DOI: 10.1097/01.BCR.0000095516.98523.04

[21] Mohammadi AA, Parand A, Kardeh S, Janati M, Mohammadi S. Efficacy of topical enalapril in the treatment of hypertrophic scars. World Journal of Plastic Surgery. 2018;**7** (3):326–331. DOI: 10.29252/wjps.7.3.326

[22] Lewis PA, Wright K, Webster A, et al. A randomized controlled pilot study comparing aqueous cream with a beeswax and herbal oil cream in the provision of relief from postburn pruritus. Journal of Burn Care & Research. 2012;**33**(4):e195–e200. DOI: 10.1097/BCR.0b013e31825042e2

[23] Baker RA, Zeller RA, Klein RL, et al. Burn wound itch control using H1 and H2 antagonists. Journal of Burn Care & Rehabilitation. 2001;**22**(4): 263–268. DOI: 10.1097/00004630-2001 07000-00003

[24] Mendham JE. Gabapentin for the treatment of itching produced by burns and wound healing in children: A pilot study. Burns. 2004;**30**(8):851–853. DOI: 10.1016/j.burns.2004.05.009

[25] Ahuja RB, Gupta R, Gupta G, Shrivastava P. A comparative analysis of cetirizine, gabapentin and their combination in the relief of post-burn pruritus. Burns. 2011;**37**(2):203–207. DOI: 10.1016/j.burns.2010.06.004

[26] Ahuja RB, Gupta GK. A four-arm, double-blind, randomized, placebo-controlled study of pregabalin in the management of post-burn pruritus. Burns. 2013;**39**(1):24–29. DOI: 10.1016/j.burns.2012.09.016

[27] Gross S, Overbaugh R, Jansen R. Ondansetron for treating itch in healing burns. Internet Journal of Pain, Symptom Control and Palliative Care. 2007;**5**(1):5–8

[28] Joo SY, Cho YS, Seo CH. The clinical utility of extracorporeal shock wave therapy for burn pruritus: A prospective, randomized, single-blind study. Burns. 2018;**44**(3):612–619. DOI: 10.1016/j.burns.2017.09.014

[29] Samhan AF, Abdelhalim NM. Impacts of low-energy extracorporeal shockwave therapy on pain, pruritus, and health-related quality of life in patients with burn: A randomized placebo-controlled study. Burns. 2019;**45**(5):1094–1101. DOI: 10.1016/j.burns.2019.02.007

[30] Allison KP, Kiernan MN, Waters RA, Clement RM. Pulsed dye laser treatment of burn scars: Alleviation or irritation? Burns. 2003;**29**(3):207–213. DOI: 10.1016/S0305-4179(02)00280-2

[31] Ebid AA, Ibrahim AR, Omar MT, El Baky AMA. Long-term effects of pulsed high-intensity laser therapy in the treatment of post-burn pruritus: A double-blind, placebo-controlled, randomized study. Lasers in Medical Science. 2017;**32**(3):693–701. DOI: 10.1007/s10103-017-2172-3

[32] Hettrick HH, O'Brien K, Laznick H, et al. Effect of transcutaneous electrical nerve stimulation for the management of burn pruritus: A pilot study. Journal of Burn Care & Rehabilitation. 2004;**25**(3):236–240. DOI: 10.1097/01.BCR.0000124745.22170.86

[33] Douglas H, Lynch J, Harms KA, et al. Carbon dioxide laser treatment in burn-related scarring: A prospective randomized controlled trial. Journal of Plastic, Reconstructive & Aesthetic Surgery. 2019;**72**(6):863–870. DOI: 10.1016/j.bjps.2019.01.027

[34] Hoseininejad SS, Rahbar R, Farhadi M, Godarzi S. Comparative evaluation of intralesional injection of botulinum toxin type A versus triamcinolone acetonide in treating post-burn pruritus. Maedica (Bucur). 2024;**19**(4):763–768. DOI: 10.26574/maedica.2024.19.4.763

[35] Cho YS, Jeon JH, Hong A, et al. The effect of burn rehabilitation massage therapy on hypertrophic scar after burn: A randomized controlled trial. Burns. 2014;**40**(8):1513–1520. DOI: 10.1016/j.burns.2014.02.005

[36] Field T, Peck M, Krugman S, Burman I, Ozment-Schenck L, et al. Postburn itching, pain, and psychological symptoms are reduced with massage therapy. Journal of Burn Care & Rehabilitation. 2000;**21**(3):189–193. DOI: 10.1067/mbc.2000.105087

[37] Spronk I, Polinder S, Haagsma JA, et al. Patient-reported scar quality of adults after burn injuries: A five-year multicenter follow-up study. Wound Repair and Regeneration. 2019;**27**(4):406–414. DOI: 10.1111/wrr.12709

[38] Gee Kee EL, Kimble RM, Cuttle L, Stockton KA. Scar outcome of children with partial thickness burns: A 3 and 6 month follow up. Burns. 2016;**42**:97–103. DOI: 10.1016/j.burns.2015.06.019

[39] Guo XY, Xie WG. (Title needed). Zhonghua Shao Shang Za Zhi. 2021;**37**(10):1000–1004. DOI: 10.3760/cma.j.cn501120-20200714-00344

[40] Sharpe JR, Booth S, Jubin K, et al. Progression of wound pH during the course of healing in burns. Journal of Burn Care & Research. 2013;**34**(3):e201–e208. DOI: 10.1097/BCR.0b013e31825d5569

[41] Preiser JC, Reper P, Vlasselaer D, et al. Nitric oxide production is increased in patients after burn injury. Journal of Trauma. 1996;**40**(3):368–371. DOI: 10.1097/00005373-199603000-00007

[42] de Chalain TM, Tang C, Thomson HG. Burn area color changes after superficial burns in childhood: Can they be predicted? Journal of Burn Care & Rehabilitation. 1998;**19**(1 Pt 1):39–49. DOI: 10.1097/00004630-199801000-00010

[43] Chadwick SL, Yip C, Ferguson MW, Shah M. Repigmentation of cutaneous scars depends on original wound type. Journal of Anatomy. 2013;**223**(1):74–82. DOI: 10.1111/joa.12052

[44] Mohamed Ali BM, Gheida SF, El Mahdy NA, Sadek SN. Evaluation of salicylic acid peeling in comparison with topical tretinoin in the treatment of postinflammatory hyperpigmentation. Journal of Cosmetic Dermatology. 2017;**16**(1):52–60. DOI: 10.1111/jocd.12301

[45] Poelchow F, Codde J, Kendell R, Edgar DW, Wood FM. A randomized investigation of film-forming silicone gel in superficial partial-thickness face and neck burn patients: Indication of improved early scar pigmentation outcomes. Burns. 2024;**50**(6):1605–1613. DOI: 10.1016/j.burns.2024.03.024

[46] Ho WS, Chan HH, Ying SY, Chan PC, Burd A, King WW. Prospective study on the treatment of postburn hyperpigmentation by intense pulsed light. Lasers in Surgery and Medicine. 2003;**32**(1):42–45. DOI: 10.1002/lsm.10139

[47] Siadat AH, Iraji F, Bahrami R, et al. Comparison between modified Kligman formulation versus Kligman formulation and intense pulsed light in the treatment of post-burn hyperpigmentation. Advanced Biomedical Research. 2016;**5**:125

[48] Wang LZ, Ding JP, Yang MY, Chen DW, Chen B. Treatment of facial post-burn hyperpigmentation using micro-plasma radiofrequency technology. Lasers in Medical Science. 2015;**30**(1):241–245. DOI: 10.1007/s10103-014-1649-6

[49] Eberlein A, Schepler H, Spilker G, Altmeyer P, Hartmann B. Erbium:YAG laser treatment of post-burn scars: Potentials and limitations. Burns. 2005;**31**(1):15–24. DOI: 10.1016/j.burns.2004.06.004

[50] Waibel J, Wulkan AJ, Lupo M, Beer K, Anderson RR. Treatment of burn scars with the 1,550 nm nonablative fractional erbium laser. Lasers in Surgery and Medicine. 2012;**44**(6):441–446. DOI: 10.1002/lsm.22038

[51] Tao J, Champlain A, Weddington C, Moy L, Tung R. Treatment of burn scars in Fitzpatrick phototype III patients using a combination of pulsed dye laser and non-ablative fractional resurfacing with 1550 nm erbium:glass/1927 nm thulium laser devices. Scars, Burns & Healing. 2018;**4**:2059513118758510. DOI: 10.1177/2059513118758510

[52] Onur Erol O, Agaoglu G, Jawad MA. Combined non-ablative laser and microfat grafting for burn scar treatment. Aesthetic Surgery Journal. 2019;**39**(4):NP55–NP67. DOI: 10.1093/asj/sjy291

[53] Moon SH, Lee SY, Jung SN, et al. Use of split thickness plantar skin grafts

in the treatment of hyperpigmented skin-grafted fingers and palms in previously burned patients. Burns. 2011;**37**(4):714–720. DOI: 10.1016/j.burns.2011.01.010

[54] Lupon E, Laloze J, Chaput B, et al. Treatment of hyperpigmentation after burn: A literature review. Burns. 2022;**48**(5):1055–1068. DOI: 10.1016/j.burns.2022.04.017

[55] Schmidt M, Serror K, Chaouat M, Mimoun M, Boccara D. Management of hypopigmented scars following burn injuries. Annales de Chirurgie Plastique Et Esthétique. 2018;**63**(3):246–254. DOI: 10.1016/j.anplas.2017.10.006

[56] Kahn AM, Cohen MJ. Treatment for depigmentation following burn injuries. Burns. 1996;**22**(7):552–554. DOI: 10.1016/0305-4179(96)88885-1

[57] Açikel C, Ulkür E, Güler MM. Treatment of burn scar depigmentation by carbon dioxide laser-assisted dermabrasion and thin skin grafting. Plastic and Reconstructive Surgery. 2000;**105**:1973–1978

[58] Harashina T, Iso R. The treatment of leukoderma after burns by a combination of dermabrasion and "chip" skin grafting. British Journal of Plastic Surgery. 1985;**38**:301–305

[59] Chen B, Xu M, Li B. Clinical experience in treating post-burn depigmentation with tiny epidermal particle grafts. International Wound Journal. 2017;**14**(1):165–171. DOI: 10.1111/iwj.12577

[60] Fujii M, Terashi H, Hashikawa K, Nomura T, Omori M, Tahara S. Thin minigrafting technique for postburn leukoderma. Dermatologic Surgery. 2007;**33**:1368–1373

[61] Busch KH, Bender R, Walezko N, Aziz H, Altintas MA, Aust MC. Combination of medical needling and non-cultured autologous skin cell transplantation (Re Nova Cell) for repigmentation of hypopigmented burn scars. Burns. 2016;**42**:1556–1566

[62] Mulekar SV, Issa AA, Eisa AA. Treatment of post-burn leucoderma with non-cultured melanocyte-keratinocyte transplantation (MKTP). Burns. 2011;**37**:448–452

[63] Dai NT, Chang HI, Wang YW, et al. Restoration of skin pigmentation after deep partial or full-thickness burn injury. Advanced Drug Delivery Reviews. 2018;**123**:155–164

[64] van der Velden EM, Baruchin AM, Jairath D, Oostrom CA, Ijsselmuiden OE. Dermatography: A method for permanent repigmentation of achromic burn scars. Burns. 1995;**21**:304–307

[65] Lupon E, Berkane Y, Bertheuil N, et al. Nonsurgical treatment of postburn hypopigmentation: A literature review. Journal of Burn Care & Research. 2024;**45**(3):601–607. DOI: 10.1093/jbcr/irae030

[66] Carney BC, McKesey JP, Rosenthal DS, Shupp JW. Treatment strategies for hypopigmentation in the context of burn hypertrophic scars. Plastic and Reconstructive Surgery Global Open. 2018;**6**(1): e1642. DOI: 10.1097/GOX.0000000000001642

[67] Calikapan GT, Akan M, Karaca M, Aköz T. Marjolin ulcer of the scalp: Intruder of a burn scar. Journal of Craniofacial Surgery. 2008;**19**(4): 1020–1025

[68] Saaiq M, Ashraf B. Marjolin's ulcers in post-burn lesions and scars. World Journal of Clinical Cases. 2014;**2**: 507–514

[69] Al-zacko SM. Malignancy in chronic burn scar: A 20-year experience in Mosul, Iraq. Burns. 2013;**39**(7): 1488–1491

[70] Enoch S, Miller D, Price P, Harding KG. Early diagnosis is vital in the management of squamous cell carcinomas associated with chronic non-healing ulcers: A case series and review of the literature. International Wound Journal. 2004;**1**(3):165–175

[71] Bazaliński D, Przybek-Mita J, Barańska B, Więch P. Marjolin's ulcer in chronic wounds-review of available literature. Contemporary Oncology (Poznan). 2017;**21**(3):197–202

[72] Sinha S, Arora R, Kutluberk E, et al. Spatial and single-cell transcriptomics reveal that oncofetal reprogramming of fibroblasts is associated with malignant degeneration of burn scar. Journal of Investigative Dermatology 2025;**145**:444–451.e11

[73] Chalya PL, Mabula JB, Rambau P, et al. Marjolin's ulcers at a University Teaching Hospital in Northwestern Tanzania: A retrospective review of 56 cases. World Journal of Surgical Oncology. 2012;**10**:38

[74] Harland DL, Robinson WA, Franklin WA. Deletion of the p53 gene in a patient with aggressive burn scar carcinoma. Journal of Trauma. 1997;**42**:104–107

[75] Hayashi M, Tamura G, Kato N, et al. Genetic analysis of cutaneous squamous cell carcinoma arising from different areas. Pathology International. 2003;**53**:602–607

[76] Pekarek B, Buck S, Osher L. A comprehensive review on Marjolin's ulcers: Diagnosis and treatment. Journal of the American College of Certified Wound Specialists. 2011;**3**:60–64

[77] Gül U, Kiliç A. Squamous cell carcinoma developing on burn scar. Annals of Plastic Surgery. 2006;**56** (4):406–408

[78] Challa VR, Deshmane V, Ashwatha Reddy MB. A retrospective study of Marjolin's ulcer over an eleven year period. Journal of Cutaneous and Aesthetic Surgery. 2014;7(3):155–159. DOI: 10.4103/0974-2077.146667

[79] Kanth AM, Heiman AJ, Nair L, et al. Current trends in the management of Marjolin's ulcer: A systematic review. Journal of Burn Care & Research. 2021;**42**(2):144–151. DOI: 10.1093/jbcr/iraa128

[80] Bozkurt M, Kapi E, Kuvat SV, et al. Current concepts in the management of Marjolin's ulcers: Outcomes from a standardized treatment protocol in 16 cases. Journal of Burn Care & Research 2010;**31**:776–780

[81] Elkins-Williams ST, Marston WA, Hultman CS. Management of the chronic burn wound. Clinics in Plastic Surgery. 2017;**44**(3):679–687. DOI: 10.1016/j.cps.2017.02.024

[82] Motamedolshariati M, Rezaei E, Beiraghi-toosi A, et al. Sentinel node mapping in Marjolin's ulcers: Is it feasible? Wounds 2015;**27**:54–62

[83] Oruç M, Kankaya Y, Sungur N, et al. Clinicopathological evaluation of

Marjolin ulcers over two decades. Kaohsiung Journal of Medical Sciences. 2017;**33**(7):327–333. DOI: 10.1016/j.kjms.2017.04.008

[84] Malheiro E, Pinto A, Choupina M. Marjolin's ulcer of the scalp: Case report and literature review. Annals of Burns and Fire Disasters. 2001;**14**:39–42

[85] Mousa AK, Elshenawy AA, Maklad SM, et al. Post-burn scar malignancy: 5-year management review and experience. International Wound Journal. 2022;**19**(4):895–909. DOI: 10.1111/iwj.13690

[86] Ozek C, Cankayali R, Bilkay U, et al. Marjolin's ulcers arising in burn scars. Journal of Burn Care & Rehabilitation. 2001;**22**:384–389

[87] Mitra S, Panda S, Sikka K, Mallick S, Thakar A. Multimodal management of locoregionally extensive Marjolin ulcer: A case report and review of the literature. Wounds. 2024;**36**(5):166–169. DOI: 10.25270/wnds/23138